Aerobatics Today

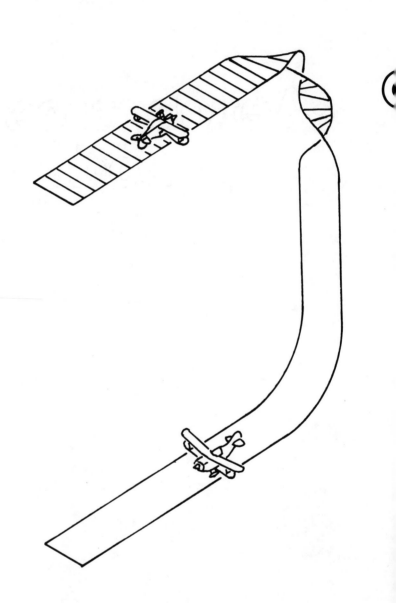

Aerobatics Today

Bob O'Dell

Revised Edition

ST. MARTIN'S PRESS
New York

Library of Congress Cataloging in Publication Data

O'Dell, Bob, 1937-
  Aerobatics today.

  1. Stunt flying.   I. Title.
GV758.033   79-25363
ISBN 0-312-00760-4

DEDICATION

For Clint McHenry, who characterizes for all of us what is meant by the words sportsman, perfectionist, gentleman.

Aerobatics Today

Foreword

Huntsville, AL 1980
THE WORDS of *Aerobatics Today* were put down by one person, but the story actually is being written by many people. Even though the book describes only a small portion of the total picture, a certain feel for the whole story should emerge from these vignettes and descriptions.

The use of the masculine notation throughout the book reflects the author's opinion that modern English does not have appropriate non-sexist terms for many situations. Many of the most enthusiastic and proficient aerobatic pilots in the United States are women: I ask them not to take umbrage.

Many persons have contributed directly and indirectly to this book: My aerobatic flight students, from whom I continuously learn; the several colleagues who have contributed facts and pictures of their aircraft; Robert Parker, who provided a critique of the section on physiology; Janice Brewer, who supported turning an idea into a text. Most of all, Betsy, Cindy and Nicholle have contributed by their patience while I have been off pursuing my own thing after building those new and better wings in the middle of the recreation room.

Houston, TX 1984

This second edition of *Aerobatics Today* has been prepared four years after the first. The changes reflect the improvements in the author's understanding of how to fly aerobatics, modifications of rules and organizations, and contributions from aerobatics competitors and enthusiasts. It is a measure of the type of people who do aerobatics that their comments on the first edition have always been constructive and often with wry good humor.

Aerobatics Today

1
Introduction

LOOKING ABOVE, you see a sky clear of clouds and deep blue; ahead it seems that you can see to the edge of the earth. Even at a height of only a few thousand feet you feel a certain isolation from the earth that you left in a tiny biplane only minutes before. The nose comes down and a feeling of acceleration touches you. With a gentle pull on the control, the airplane leaps upward, pointed straight for the sky. Suddenly you feel absolutely alone, free, and independent as you are carried higher and higher, approaching the feeling known only by those few who have actually left this green earth. At last, when the earth's gravity has gently slowed your upward rush and you pause motionless, briefly suspended in space, you quickly push the rudder control and the blue sky is replaced with the early summer green and lines of field and pasture. Now the pull of the earth makes itself felt fully as you gain speed in a downward rush. A second pull on the control and you again weigh many times your normal weight. You are pressed into your seat and the parachute harness that encloses you and soon you are back to level. The earth and sky are the same, the machine is no different, but you are. You have truly slipped the bonds of earth, if only briefly, and this experience cannot be erased.

The description above is not of a rare experience shared by only a mystic few, but describes a simple aerobatic maneuver as flown by an increasing number of enthusiasts throughout the world. Aerobatics have been with us almost as long as powered flight, but in the past few years the activity has grown from the isolated pursuit of a few sportsmen and "flying fools" into an art pursued by thousands of pilots.

At many small airports throughout the United States, weekends find men and women building, servicing and, most of all, flying a special breed of machine, the aerobatic airplane. In this machine they find a deep sense of personal satisfaction and endless challenge. The skills needed are first learned with someone else, then brought to perfection alone, eventually leading to individual exploration and learning. Those skills are often tested by weekend gatherings where pilots fly alone in front of trained judges. Not all of these tests are weekend affairs. There is a national competition when hundreds come together not only to strive for recognition and award but also to share experiences and enjoy the companionship of others with common goals and interests. This is the picture in aerobatics today, and one that will be described in this book.

This book is written for three types of readers: pilots, flying enthusiasts and everyone else, whom we'll call laymen. There should be something in it for each of these groups relevant to their backgrounds and their view of the sport of aerobatics.

Those of you who are pilots should find something here; you will appreciate that being an aviator means continuously learning, and the type of flying skills acquired in aerobatics is different from what you have been taught. In today's aviation training, the emphasis is on learning to fly specific sets of training maneuvers in training airplanes, with the emphasis on how the examining federal agency says a maneuver should be executed in a flight test. Genuinely understanding how an air machine works seems secondary in the modern student pilot's course syllabus, whereas the final examination performance seems paramount. Pilots trained in this fashion are not prepared for the many possible conditions they can encounter. It is a wise pilot who appreciates the need to learn about aerobatic flying in order to illuminate some of those dark corners left in his early formal training. Some of you pilots will be happy to read about it, while others will be satisfied with enough of a sample to say that you know what it is really like. Others of you may feel that aerobatics is something that you'd like to do, but did not quite know how to get started. This book should help.

Flying enthusiasts far outnumber licensed pilots, and those who fall in this group should appreciate armchair aerobatics as much as any reader. For reasons of health, wealth or other circumstance, this may be the only type of flying available to you. It is a way of going flying that is independent of time or weather and can be the next best thing to being there. Perhaps this book will help you find some way of sampling the pleasure flying really offers.

Laymen outnumber us all, and you are probably interested in all aspects of life in our modern society. The aviation industry touches the lives of most modern Americans, and you will probably want to know about a pursuit followed by many, including many of those who sit up in the front office of airliners. The airliner is not flown by an impersonal voice that settles you in and tells you how long it's going to take to get to your destination. Rather, it is flown by a team of individuals, with individual skills and experiences. The airline passenger should feel far more comfortable knowing there is a disciplined pilot up front who has encountered flight in all its aspects and who is its master. Finally, there may be the amateur sociologists and psychologists who are interested in a rapidly growing recreational field and want to understand why others pursue the sport. When George Mallory answered the question of why he wanted to climb Mt. Everest with "Because it is there," he puzzled a lot of readers. The same type of question can be asked about aerobatic flying, and the answer is equally difficult to state. Perhaps this book will give the reasons to readers, even if, at the end, they too are unable to give an acceptable one-line response.

This book has three major parts. There is no division into sections, and the boundaries may not be all that clear when reading continuously from chapter to chapter. However, it should be something like crossing the Mason-Dixon line; there may not be any signposts, but once you're into the new territory, you'll know the difference. The first parts deal with getting started in aerobatics in terms of equipment, preparation and rules. The most intensive parts focus on the maneuvers that constitute aerobatics. The intent here is to allow the reader to understand aerobatic maneuvers and how they are flown. It is not intended to be a primer from which to teach or to teach oneself. Some maneuvers, for example, the Barrel Roll, can be done in many ways. In all cases, we'll discuss how they are flown according to international criteria, as laid out by the International Aerobatic Club, the leading aerobatic organization in the United States. Finally, we'll discuss how aerobatic flying is organized in terms of club activities and competition flying. The best aerobatic flying ever done is being done right now, and it is possible to share in this, as a pilot, judge or enthusiast. We'll discuss how.

WHY DO AEROBATICS?

Aerobatic flying is the purest form of flying—done only for personal satisfaction. It is not done to travel from one place to the other, to make a living or to bolster the defense of a country; rather, it is done for the pleasure of the doing and what it brings to us individually. While leading to this personal goal, aerobatics also meets some more specific needs.

Aerobatic flying gives the pilot a depth of knowledge that can be applied in many circumstances. The number of incidents when light aircraft are caught in the turbulence generated by a landing airliner increases every year. These situations sometimes end tragically, for the average pilot has never seen the world while the plane is on its wing tip or inverted, and being introduced to this angle at low altitude often leads to the wrong corrective action. Stall-spin accidents are still one of the biggest killers, accounting for 20 to 25 percent of the fatalities among general aviation pilots. Spins are not required for any pilot license until the Certified Flight Instructor rating; and even then, it is only required that dual instruction in Spins has been received. It is incredible to think of such an elementary maneuver being such a widespread killer, but it is, largely because the first time an average pilot encounters a Spin he does so accidentally. Often this first introduction is the last, but a large number of the survivors then wisely obtain dual instruction on Spins as soon as they can. The ability to recover rapidly from an unusual attitude or from a Spin is one of the most important parts of a pilot's training, and aerobatics are the best way to acquire the ability.

Not only is the aerobatic pilot safer, he is also more efficient. He knows the operating limitations of his machine and how to get the best performance from it. Maximum rates of climb, coordination of control use and speed control are all natural to the aerobatic pilot. These skills are called for even when flying non-aerobatic airplanes, giving greater efficiency and fuel economy in flying.

In our modern society, the frontiers seem to be contracting. There is no unfilled continent lying before us, drawing the adventurous to its boundaries. The basic drive that leads to exploration is still there in all of us and is quite strong in many. Aerobatics can be a natural outlet for this drive, for it is an endless challenge and one that is ultimately met alone. Alone, but with oneself, and there is no better way of getting to know yourself and to come to terms with that person.

WHAT ARE AEROBATICS?

So far we've talked a lot about aerobatics but haven't paused long enough to make sure that we're talking about the same thing. A safe place to start is with Webster's *New 20th-Century Dictionary of the English Language:*

> aer·o·bat·ics 1. Spectacular feats done in flying as loops, rolls, etc.
> 2. The art of doing such feats in flying.

The legal definition given by Federal Aviation Regulations (Part 91.71) is less poetic: "An abrupt change in attitude, an abnormal attitude or abnormal acceleration not necessary for normal flight." One man's normal may be another's abnormal, so this "legal" definition only helps a little. A more quantitative statement intended to apply to aerobatics is Federal Aviation Regulation 91.15, which requires parachutes for flight at bank angles of more than 60° and nose-up or nose-down attitudes of more than 30° from the horizon.

The term *aerobatics* is used widely, but not by our regulating agency, the Federal Aviation Administration (the FAA). They still use the term *acrobatics* instead of *aerobatics.* Since *acrobatics* brings up mental pictures of a circus ring filled with over-developed men and women in sequins and tight clothes performing their versions of "spectacular feats," it is a term not used by devotees of the sport. Although as long as the FAA continues to be positive in their general policy towards aerobatics, we probably shouldn't complain about what they call it.

There is one thing that aerobatics is not, and this must be emphasized. Aerobatics is *not* stunt flying. Stunt flying started very early in aviation, probably the first time a pilot climbed into an air machine to get someone else's attention because he couldn't get that notice in any other way. This type of flying continues today, but it has no place in serious aerobatics. Stunt flying requires little skill and lots of disregard for others.

This book is heavily oriented toward private and competition aerobatics, ignoring the well-known area of airshow flying. Airshow flying is an important part of publicizing flying for the public, but is a mixed bag. Some of the best aerobatic pilots do airshows, while some of the "ace" airshow pilots couldn't make the upper half at a regional aerobatic competition. There is a certain analogy with television wrestling as contrasted with competition wrestling. In both cases, the money is good; that is the attraction.

This book is unapologetically intended to cover American aerobatics. This scene is quite broad enough for description apart from the activity in other nations. The legal rules cited will be those applying within the United States and may differ from those in other nations. The aircraft used as examples are of American manufacture because these are the airplanes that most of the readers will see and fly. Since the sense of rotation of American aircraft engines is not necessarily the same as those built in other countries, in some cases the correction for engine effects such as engine torque may not work in the direction indicated. In each such case, we try to work from basic principles, and the foreign reader can make the necessary translations.

2
Aerobatic Aircraft— State of the Art

MORE AND BETTER aerobatic aircraft are being built today than ever before. These aircraft vary from simple modifications of basic trainers to snarling, specialized competition machines. Some of these attract no more attention at the local airport than an idle question about why that airplane has checkerboards on its tail. Others attract a crowd wherever they go because they exude strength and performance. The important thing here is that aerobatic aircraft of a variety of types are widely available and there is at least one within the financial and skill capabilities of all pilots.

Early aerobatic flying was dominated by the many designs developed for military training and use. This was largely because of their availability and strength and not because they were all that suited for aerobatics. Any airplane design represents a compromise among many, sometimes conflicting, goals, and it should come as no surprise that the best aerobatic airplanes start with aerobatic capability as their paramount goal.

8

The military demonstration teams are impressive in their skill and precision, while their aircraft have impressive speed and sound levels, but the small aerobatic airplane has a far bigger repertory. The propeller-driven aerobatic airplane is being improved continuously, and some maneuvers being done today were impossible by yesterday's standards. Never before have aerobatic aircraft been so widely available.

WHAT IS AN AEROBATIC AIRCRAFT?

If we are to talk about aerobatic aircraft, we need to know what they are and what sets them apart. Whether we are considering assembly line or home-built aircraft, the same basic considerations apply, even though the formal governing regulations differ. The most important factors are structural strength, freedom from adverse control characteristics and aerodynamic performance. There are many aircraft in which a skilled pilot can perform maneuvers that satisfy the FAA's definition of an aerobatic maneuver; however, the structural safety margin is small. The true safety margin depends critically upon the experience and skill of the pilot and is never very great. For an airplane to be truly safe for aerobatics, it must demonstrate by design, construction and performance that it can do certain types of maneuvers with an ample safety margin.

Structural strength is measured in terms of the load factor. Load factor is the ratio of the apparent weight of the aircraft to its true weight. Load factors result from moving the aircraft in a direction different from that favored by its momentum. We experience a load factor of one, also called one G, in straight and level flight. When we turn the airplane rapidly or rapidly change to a high angle of attack, we experience a higher load factor because the airplane's momentum is straight ahead. A "top of the roller coaster" sensation comes from abrupt changes to downward flight and are associated with negative load factors. High positive and negative load factors—whether from intentional or unintentional maneuvers—can cause an aircraft to bear an apparent weight far in excess of its design strength. Aerobatic aircraft are designed with limit load factors of plus six and at least minus three G's, which means that this range of values can be experienced without structural damage. This range is ample for almost all circumstances. Beyond the limit load factor, up to 50 percent more, the aircraft will possibly sustain permanent damage. Beyond this range (plus nine and minus six G's), the aircraft may break up.

Control characteristics are important since control surface flutter, especially in the ailerons, has been encountered in many aircraft designs when flown at high speeds, sometimes with tragic results. The aerobatic aircraft must show itself to be free of such flutter over its operating speed range. Likewise, it must have controls that are effective at all speeds encountered.

Finally, when we define an aerobatic aircraft, we must consider the factors loosely grouped under the term *aerodynamic performance.* Aerodynamic performance, which is not a legal term, includes such factors as stall speed, maximum level flight speed, rate of roll and rate of climb. Once the safety considerations of load factors and freedom from flutter are met, it is these characteristics that will largely determine the performance characteristics of an aerobatic aircraft.

A low stall speed means the ability to fly off the top of certain climbing maneuvers, while a high maximum speed means longer up lines and larger loops, giving more time to execute additional maneuvers. Rate of climb is also a measure of expected vertical performance and the size of maneuvers.

These characteristics are both important and easy to determine for any aircraft, but the same cannot be said for the roll rate. Even for the same aircraft, various roll rates are often quoted, sometimes owing to the difficulty of measuring this quantity, but often the result of a certain amount of thrown in halo effect. A useful measure of expected approximate rate of roll will be the ratio of the maximum level flight velocity to the wingspan. As an approximation, all airplanes of similar design will roll faster at higher airspeeds, while airplanes with shorter wingspans roll faster at a given airspeed. Another way of saying this is that: given two similar airplanes flying at the same speed, the one with the smaller wingspan will roll faster. Also, a given airplane will roll faster at higher speeds.

AVAILABLE AEROBATIC AIRCRAFT

Now that we know what legal and practical characteristics define an aerobatic aircraft, let's have a look at what aircraft are available. The lists given here will be relatively short and will irritate at least a few people since *their* favorite may not be included. What I have intended is to include the most popular aircraft that have established themselves as training or competition machines. For legal purposes there are two types of aerobatic aircraft, the Certificated Aircraft and the Experimental Aircraft. The designations of "manufactured" and "custom built" are more descriptive although not recognized in any legal sense.

Manufactured (Certificated) aircraft are those aircraft that have proved to the FAA by design, analysis and performance that they are able to satisfy the legal requirements of an aerobatic aircraft and that have demonstrated the ability to do aerobatics. The specific maneuvers allowed are entered in the operating manual. These aircraft are manufactured under close quality control and are subject to the maintenance regulations of all manufactured aircraft. Changes between models and the temperaments of previous owners and mechanics notwithstanding, a well-maintained model of a given manufactured aircraft represents a fairly well-defined set of performance characteristics.

Table 1 gives a selected list of manufactured aircraft and the most important characteristics for describing the expected aerobatic performance. This alphabetical list includes only those now or recently in production. The first four are closed cabin, the last three are open cockpit, although the Pitts' have optional bubble canopies. The list includes basic trainers and beginning competition machines (Aerobat and Citabria), intermediate trainers and competitors (CAP–10, Decathlon, Great Lakes), and a very high performance machine (Pitts S1S). The two-place Pitts (S2A) occupies a place just below the single place (S1S) in performance but has the advantage of room for a passenger or instructor. All these aircraft are seen frequently in the United States except the CAP-10, which is of French manufacture. Because the CAP-10 has made its mark in our national competition and is available in the United States, it certainly deserves inclusion here. All these aircraft are available through the manufacturers and their dealers and used models are widely advertised in trade publications such as *Trade-A-Plane* (Crossville, TN 38555).

Custom-built (Experimental) aircraft do not have the pedigree of the manufactured aircraft, having been built by individuals or small groups. As in other situations, the lack of a pedigree (certification) does not indicate a lack of performance, safety or quality. Indeed, it is likely the best workmanship and performance will be found among these aircraft, since the private builder does not have to pay for his labor (himself). The custom-built aircraft do show greater variation in performance and workmanship within a given type than the manufactured aircraft. This is because their construction is by individuals working on one airplane at a time, and they are maintained by different procedures.

The custom-built aircraft listed in Table 2 are, for the most part, designs that have been built by numerous individuals, have flown for several years and have proven themselves as

TABLE 1 MANUFACTURED AEROBATIC AIRCRAFT

	Aerobat[1]	CAP-10[2]	Citabria[3]	Decathlon[3]	Pitts S1S[4]	Pitts S1T[4]	Pitts S2A[4]	Pitts S2S[4]	Pitts S2B[4]
Seats	Two	Two	Two	Two	One	One	Two	One	Two
Wings	One	One	One	One	Two	Two	Two	Two	Two
Gross Weight (Aero) (lbs.)	1670	1675	1650	1800	1150	1150	1500	1500	1700
Power (hp)	110	180	115–150	150–180	180	200	200	260	260
Propeller[5]	FP	FP	FP	FP-CS	FP	CS	CS	CS	CS
Wingspan (ft.)	33.2	26.4	33.4	32	17.3	17.3	20.0	20.0	20.0
Wing Loading (lbs/ft²)	10.5	14.3	10.0	11.3	11.7	11.7	12.0	12.0	13.6
Power Loading (lbs/hp)	15.2	9.3	14.3	12.0–10.0	6.4	5.8	7.5	5.8	6.5
Stall Speed (mph)	56 (w/o flaps)	58 (w/o flaps)	51	54	61	64	62	58	60
Top Speed (mph)	125	170	125–132	142–148	[6]146	185	165	187	187
Rate of Climb (fpm)[7]	715	1600	725–1120	880–1230	2500	2800	1900	2800	2700
Top Speed/Wingspan (mph/ft)	3.8	6.4	3.7–4.0	4.4–4.6	[7]8.4	10.7	8.25	9.4	9.4
Inverted Systems	No	Yes	No-Yes	Yes	Yes	Yes	Yes	Yes	Yes

[1]Cessna Aircraft Co., Wichita, KS 67201; side by side seating.
[2]Mudry Aviation Ltd., Dutchess County Airport/Wappinger Falls, NY 12590; side by side seating.
[3]No longer manufactured, but many almost new aircraft are still available.
[4]Pitts Aerobatics, P. O. Box 547, Afton, WY 83110.
[5]Fixed Pitch (FP) or Constant Speed (CS)
[6]Cruise Power limited by engine redline.
[7]Sea level values

aerobatic performers. There are many other designs flying, although not as widely available on the market as these.

The Clipped Wing Cubs and Taylorcraft are modifications of two venerable light aircraft. The conversions involve shortening the wings to increase the roll rate, strengthening the airframe and wings and (often) installing higher-horsepower power plants and propellers. Sometimes even inverted fuel and oil systems are added. Their low operating speeds set them in a class apart from most other aerobatic aircraft, a class which needs no apologies as they are versatile, impressive performers.

The Skybolt and Starduster Too are both two-place biplanes that are becoming increasingly popular and available. They are good performers through intermediate level maneuvers and offer the opportunity for the panache of open cockpit aerobatics for two.

The Pitts Special (S1S) is probably the most popular aerobatic design. Today's airplane is a straightforward growth from the original design of the early 1940's by Curtis Pitts, which had two ailerons, M-6 airfoil (nearly flat bottom) wings and 90 horsepower. Now most new Pitts are built with four ailerons (like the other biplanes in the table), symmetric airfoil wings and 180 horsepower. This is the aircraft used by the entire United States National Team, which won the world championship in France in 1972, and remains the most common competition mount.

The Stephens Akro is a high-performance monoplane which operates at higher speeds than the higher drag biplanes and uses its greater speeds to produce excellent roll rates and vertical penetrations. Its greater size makes it easy to see, a benefit when you are flying well. This is the basic aircraft used by Leo Loudenslager in developing his Laser-200, in which he won the United States National Championship seven times between 1975 and 1982.

Loudenslager is now working with Christen Industries, Inc. in developing a new, advanced technology aircraft based on the

TABLE 2 CUSTOM BUILT AIRCRAFT

	Clipped Wing Cub[2]	Clipped Wing Taylorcraft[3]	Eagle II[4]	Pitts S1S[5]	Skybolt[6]	Starduster Too[7]	Stephens Akro[8]
Seats	One (aero.) Two (X-Country)	One (aero.) Two (X-Country)	Two	One	Two	Two	One
Wings	One	One	Two	Two	Two	Two	One
Gross Weight (lbs)	1100	1500 (1250 aero.)	1578 (1290 competition)	1150	1750	1710	1250
Power (hp)	90	150	200	180	200	180	200
Propeller	FP	FP	CS	FP	CS	CS	FP
Wingspan (ft)	28	27.5	20	17.3	24	24	24.5
Wing Loading (lbs/ft^2)	6.7	8.9 (aero.)	10.3 (comp.)	11.7	11.7	10.4	12.8
Power Loading (lbs/hp)	12.2	8.5 (aero.)	6.5 (comp.)	6.4	8.8	9.5	6.25
Stall Speed (mph)	46	42	58	61	59	56	67
Top Speed (mph)	103	140	184	167	139	137	175
Rate of Climb (fpm)	730	1200	2100	2500	1250	1150	2700
Top Speed/Wingspan	3.7	5.1	9.2	9.7	5.8	5.8	7.1

[1] Performance characteristics values taken from actual aircraft. Design characteristics may vary with individual builders.
[2] Wag-Aero, P. O. Box 181, 1216 North Road, Lyons, WI 53148.
[3] Swick Aircraft Corp., Rt. 1, Box 203, McKinney, TX 75069.
[4] Christen Industries, Inc., 1048 Santa Ana Valley Road, Hollister, CA 95023. Certificated versions of this aircraft and a 260 horsepower stablemate will be available soon.
[5] Pitts Aerobatics, P.O. Box 547, Afton, WY 83110. Several of the Pitts designs are available for custom builders.
[6] Steen Aero Lab, 15623 De Gaulle Cir., Brighton, CO 80601.
[7] Stolp Starduster Corp., 4301 Twining, Riverside, CA 92509.
[8] G. M. Zimmerman, 8563 W. 68th Place, Arvada, CO 80002.

experience with his Laser, to be called the Laser 260. This aircraft will feature use of modern composite materials and a 260 horsepower engine.

The established position of the 180-horsepower Pitts S1S does not go unchallenged. Almost annually we hear of the newest specialized aircraft that is going to blow the Pitts out of competition. Some of these designs attain their full performance and just don't measure up in competition, while others experience unexpected difficulties in development.

The extra performance achieved by a number of customized variations of the Pitts S1S and Stephens Akro designs means that more performance can be built into these basic approaches. We see this best in the highly modified versions that were used by the United States National Teams in the 1978 through 1984 world competitions, where all of the aircraft were modified versions of these two approaches, and the modifications paid off in higher performance.

When we look at this total list, we see that there are a wide variety of aircraft available to the aerobatic pilot. Some will be found on the rental line at airports, others at aerobatic schools. Some are owned only by clubs or private owners. Aerobatic aircraft constitute only a small fraction of the total number of light aircraft, but there are enough choices that if you are interested in aerobatics, you will undoubtedly be able to find an aircraft not far from your needs.

It must be remembered that in spite of its origins and reputation, its nameplate and license, a given airplane may not be a safe aerobatic aircraft. Each machine must have its basic integrity confirmed by close inspection and must be maintained thoroughly. What has been given in this chapter should be used as a guide to what is generally available. In the final analysis, it is up to the pilot to determine that he is flying a safe aircraft each and every day that he flies.

THE BEST AEROBATIC AIRCRAFT

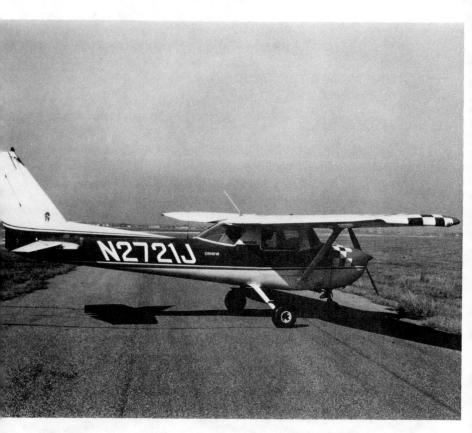

The Cessna 152 Aerobat is a popular basic trainer for many of the primary maneuvers.

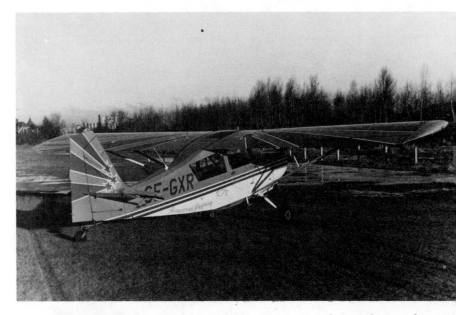

The Bellanca Decathlon is a tandem seat manufactured aircraft capable of upright and inverted flight.
Photo courtesy of Olle Vossman.

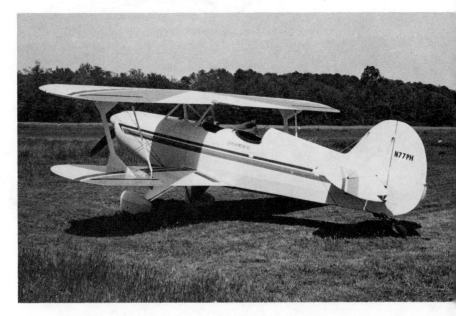

The Steen Skybolt is a two-seat custom-built aircraft that can accept a variety of engines. It offers open cockpit flying at its best.

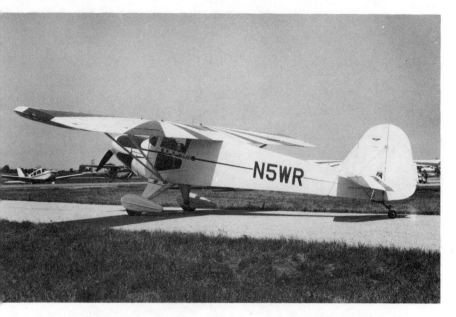

The Clipped Wing Taylorcraft is a modified, strengthened version of a venerable aircraft. In its modified form it is considered a custom-built aircraft.

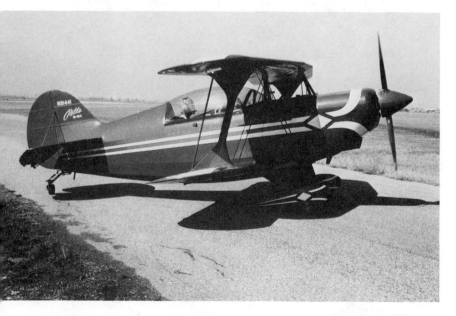

The Pitts S2A is a high-performance two-seat manufactured aircraft, offering the chance for dual instruction in the most advanced maneuvers.

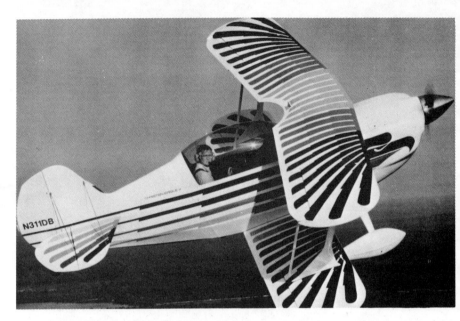

The Christen Eagle II is a quality two-place custom-built aircraft that has gained wide popularity.
Photo courtesy of Dick Blair.

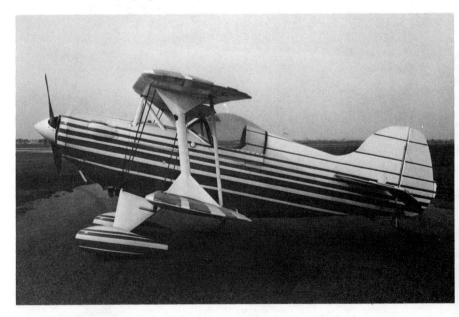

The single place Pitts S1S is the original aircraft in the wide lines of Pitts aircraft. It remains the standard for comparison.

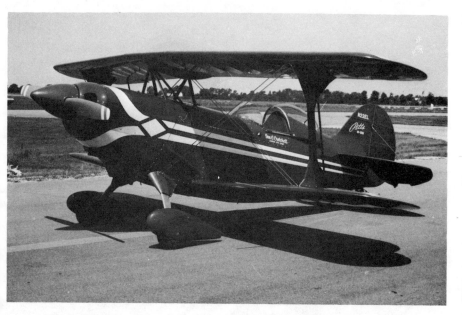

The 260 horsepower, single-place Pitts S2S offers a nice combination of high performance and excellent visibility from the ground.

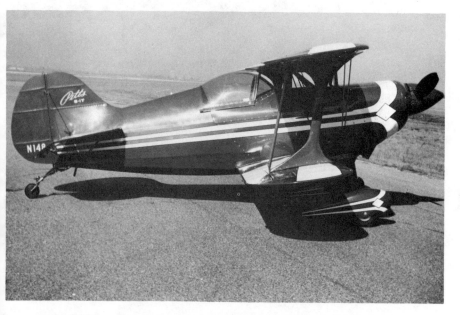

The 220 horsepower, constant speed propeller Pitts S1T packs the greatest performance per pound of the manufactured aircraft. Although closely resembling the S1S, it is a re-engineered design.

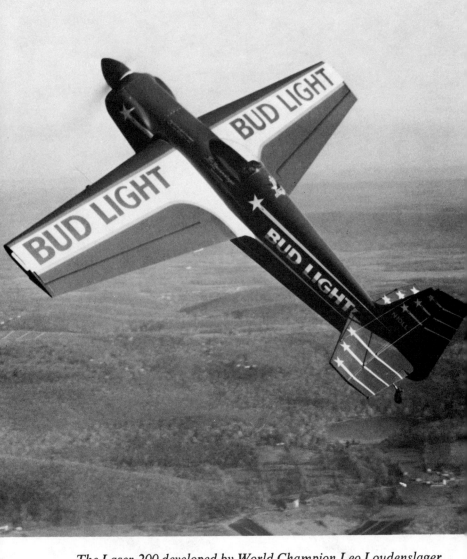

The Laser-200 developed by World Champion Leo Loudenslager is considered the top of the line among many aerobatic competitors.
Photo courtesy of Leo Loudenslager.

3
Rules—Common Sense and Legal

THE WORD *rules* can be an ugly one, especially when there are so many regulations as to make you feel your freedom is restricted. It might seem to some that the type of pilot who pursues aerobatics would not be the rule-observing type, but this is not the case. Aerobatic flying requires self-discipline, and there are many rules that *must* be observed if you are to return to fly another day. Fortunately, few of these rules are written into legal regulations. The code of conduct is largely established through common knowledge among the initiated and observed because these people want to comply and need to do so. Some rules exist to protect ourselves, our passengers and the public; others exist to protect the good image of aerobatics and to prevent the making of laws to govern this activity. Laws of restriction have a way of being made, but never rescinded. It is better to make and observe our own, thus avoiding a group of strangers doing it for us.

This chapter will address the rules that govern aerobatic

17

flight, both those that appear within the Federal Aviation Regulations and those that do not. These rules fall into four areas, covering the questions: What equipment is needed? Where can I do aerobatics? Under what conditions can aerobatics be done? Who can do aerobatics?

AIRCRAFT

The previous chapter describes a number of aircraft types that are usually considered aerobatic, but concludes with the important admonition that a nameplate alone does not make any particular aircraft safe for aerobatics. The manufactured aircraft is designed with certain structural strengths. Controlled manufacturing techniques are then relied upon to guarantee that others of its type have the same properties. The prototypes of these aircraft are thoroughly tested in the air, and it is determined which maneuvers can safely be executed. This set of maneuvers becomes part of that airplane's operating manual and are usually listed in a placard in the cockpit, together with recommended entry speeds. Very few aerobatic aircraft are unrestricted and the established repertoire of maneuvers must be observed if the aircraft is to be operated safely and legally. Fatal accident reports and bent airplanes sitting in service hangars (being made straight by large applications of money) attest to the wisdom of observing the list of approved maneuvers.

The fact that a nameplate and general appearance don't make an airplane safe is emphasized by the recent case of a former military trainer. The appearance of this aircraft, a T28, oozes STRENGTH and indeed, the type makes an excellent advanced trainer for aerobatics. The owner of this particular one did not pay attention to the fact that when the wings were slightly lengthened its operating limitations had been changed to exclude aerobatics. The pilot and an unknowing passenger paid the ultimate penalty when the wings and then the tail separated in midair during a simple loop. There are lots of safe manufactured aircraft—make sure that you use one of them.

Since custom-built aircraft are not built under conditions of strict supervision, the legal performance capabilities are determined for each individual aircraft and are specified in the operating limitations issued by an FAA inspector, who will consider the design and construction of the aircraft and the results of a demonstration flight. The particular way in which the regulation is observed varies among individual inspectors and General Aviation District Offices (the level at which these tests are administered). Some operating limitations give characteristic maneuvers which establish safe flight regimes, while others require demonstration and testing of every individual maneuver. If there are no aerobatic maneuvers on the operating limitations of a custom-built aircraft, none can legally be performed.

The International Aerobatic Club places additional requirements on custom-built aircraft used in their competitions. These requirements include installation of dual lap belts and single shoulder harness, and a flight demonstration of a load factor of six. These requirements make sense for anyone considering use of a custom-built aircraft.

Whichever type of aerobatic mount you use, it is essential that you understand how it works, especially the fuel and oil systems. This is particularly true of aircraft with inverted fuel and oil supplies, where there are more parts to fail, in new and extraordinary ways. They probably won't, but you should know the systems well enough to know what to watch out for and what to do in the event of a problem.

PARACHUTES

Federal Aviation Regulations [91.15(c)] require that the pilot and all passengers wear a parachute while aerobatics are being

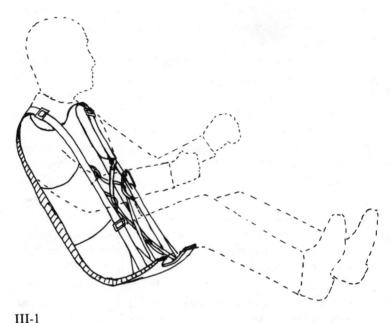

III-1

The modern thin pack parachute is comfortable when the pilot is seated and takes up little space inside the cockpit (after Security Parachute Company).

performed. Law does not require parachutes for solo aerobatics, under a general philosophy that endangering others is to be avoided but personal risk is acceptable. Lack of legal requirements aside: WEAR A PARACHUTE AT ALL TIMES WHEN DOING AEROBATICS! There are a number of pilots walking around today because of this extra-legal but common sense rule. They are easy to pick out—they smile a lot.

Parachutes are licensed safety devices, built under specific regulations and cannot legally be used unless they are "within pack." This means that back-pack parachutes must have been inspected and repacked within the last 120 days, seat-pack parachutes within the last 60 days. There are several new slim, lightweight parachutes now on the market, with the Security model being the most popular. In this case, the canopy is stored both along the back and under the buttocks, so that a 60-day repack cycle normally applies. Members of the International Aerobatic Club have been included in a special waiver allowing 120 day cycles on these parachutes for the past several years. However, this is an annual waiver and should be checked each year.

SURVIVAL

The primary elements in safety are good training, flying skill and good judgment, but you must observe other things while these capabilities are being acquired and even after.

Seatbelts are a must for all flying, and dual seatbelts are prudent in an aerobatic aircraft. Brief periods of negative G are not uncommon in even the elementary trainers and an accidentally unhooked lap belt can produce a big surprise in a closed cabin aircraft, not to mention what can happen in an open cockpit! The second belt can't hurt in the event of a sudden deceleration (crash), but dual belts are of most use while in the air.

A shoulder harness is a must too, but be sure that it is installed properly. It is of most use on the ground in the event of an unmentionable, that is, a sudden unplanned deceleration. Its purpose is to keep your upper body and head off the instrument panel and windshield, and it will only do this effectively if the shoulder harness attaches high on the airframe, at least as high as your shoulders and preferably above. A properly attached shoulder harness will not only restrain forward mo-

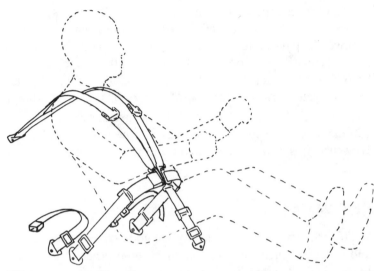

III-2

The complete aerobatic seatbelt harness includes a lapbelt, shoulder straps and a crotch strap, which shares the negative G load. A backup lapbelt finishes the complement (after Christen Industries, Inc.).

tion but will also prevent compression damage to the vertebrae, which can result if a shoulder harness is attached too low. During negative G flight, the shoulder harness should not be so tight that it carries your weight, a situation that is both uncomfortable and restricts your circulation. In inverted flight the lap belts should carry your weight and they should be tight. A crotch strap is the best way of carrying the inverted flight load.

All parachutes restrict movement to some degree. It is important that satisfying the parachute requirement does not prevent you from being able to leave the airplane in a big hurry!

A final survival rule also deals with a procedure: preflight inspection. This is a must for all aircraft but the preflight inspection is even more important for the aerobatic aircraft. These airplanes are worked hard and close to their structural limitations. This means that the aircraft must be inspected as if your life depended on it. It does. The power train becomes a region of thorough study instead of just a place to check the oil and feel the propeller for nicks. The wings are appendages to be examined for broken ribs and telltale wrinkles in the fabric, wrinkles that tell you something inside has changed. Finally, the tail group is explored for damage and the inside inspected for foreign bodies. Everything loose ends up snuggled against the rudder post in a tailwheel airplane, and many cases of control blockage in flight result from such sliding. At an early aerobatic competition, one older and wiser contest official took his flashlight and inspected the tail section of all the aircraft, each of which had been inspected by the pilot "only last week." He filled a small cardboard box with maps, handkerchiefs, tools and missing hardware!

MISCELLANEOUS

In addition to the major equipment items I have mentioned, there are a few other things that are also worth including when you fly. A G meter is valuable not only as a safety record of the conditions to which your airplane has been exposed, but also as a training aid. The G meter is simply a compact recording scale. This scale measures the effective weight of a piece of metal and displays this weight in terms of its weight under one gravity. If it weighs two pounds on the ground and 10 pounds at the entry to a Hammerhead, then five G's would be shown. As the aircraft turns and changes direction in pitch, the load factor on the airframe varies and the G meter continuously indicates this variation. Most G meters are of the recording type: the pointer pushes a pair of friction-loaded needles ahead of it in both directions. This means that the recording needles stay behind at the maximum excursion G values. Therefore, when flying away after doing a maneuver such as an inside-outside Cuban Eight, in which loads of plus three to minus three G's and all values in between are encountered, the G

THE G METER

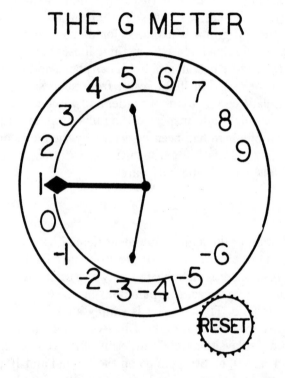

III-3

The G meter tells the pilot what the G load is at any instant, and also records the maximum and minimum values that have been experienced.

meter pointer would read 1 G (level upright flight) and +3 and −3 would be recorded on the friction needles. These needles are reset by a knob on the front of the instrument to the recording needle value.

Two personal items conclude our list of equipment: eyeglass holders and earplugs. The novice pilot often discovers at his first exposure to even mild negative G forces that eyeglasses are fitted only for positive G conditions. This could be disconcerting if you got into this position accidentally and needed those spectacles to navigate. Special elastic bands (sold in sporting goods stores) will do the job nicely, even under high negative G forces.

Earplugs are optional in lower-power aircraft, but become a necessity in high-power and performance competition machines. A 110-horsepower Cessna Aerobat produces a noise level of about 95 decibels at cruise; a 150-horsepower Decathlon, about 100 decibels at cruise, while a 180-horsepower closed canopy Pitts S1S produces a level of about 113 decibels. United States Department of Labor regulations limit daily exposure to 15 minutes at 115 decibels, 30 minutes at 110, one hour at 105, two hours at 100, and so on. Ear protection is a must if one is to avoid the risk of permanent hearing loss. As long as your ear protection does not mute too much sound, you should still be able to hear all those clues about the engine and airplane.

WHERE AEROBATICS CAN BE DONE

Two principal restrictions apply here: location and altitude. We'll address these in turn, starting with location.

Federal Aviation Regulations (91.71) forbids aerobatic flight over any congested area of a city, town or settlement, over an open air assembly of persons or within a control zone or Federal Airway. These regulations make sense and must be observed if one is to avoid endangering persons on the ground and in the air. The swivel-neck procedure taught to student pilots really finds its application in aerobatics where rapid changes of direction and altitude are the rule and not the exception.

A few other common sense rules apply to location. It is well stated that one man's music is another man's noise. The sweet sound of an aircraft engine doing what it was built to do may be an irritant to someone living close to your usual practice area. This can be especially true if you like seeing the sun come up from the top of a hammerhead on Sunday mornings and that's his time for catching up on sleep. A good-neighbor policy doesn't hurt, and ruffled feathers are easier to avoid than to smooth.

It is a fact of life that airplanes used for aerobatics give their pilots reason to land in a hurry more frequently than aircraft engaged in cross-country flight. We do everything we can to prevent the need for sudden landings, but we also must prepare for that quick trip to the ground. We may need to figure out what that change in sound or control feel means or even why there isn't any fuel flowing to the engine. To best prepare for this emergency, use a standard practice area over a place where the plane can be landed without incident. This can be a field you've checked out, a spray plane grass strip or even the local small airport, although you should keep your practice altitude well up above the traffic pattern. Some preplanning here can avoid risking a beautiful and expensive machine because of a minor mechanical problem.

Altitude is the single most important factor in safely performing aerobatics. Federal Aviation Regulations give a minimum altitude above the terrain of 1500 feet; it is just that, a minimum. A muffed maneuver, followed by a dive to high speed or a multiple turn spin can quickly use up an impressive amount of altitude, which cannot be replaced when you need it most. Novice aerobatic pilots need to have an extra margin of altitude, for their mistakes will be more frequent and their recover-

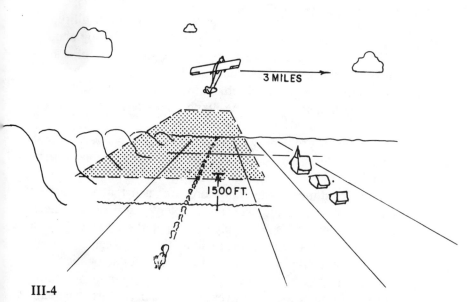

III-4

Aerobatics can be done in many places, but any one place must satisfy all the relevant Federal Aviation Regulations. The primary ones deal with minimum altitude, visibility and avoidance of congested areas.

ies will use up more altitude. Even the prudent experienced pilot adds additional altitude for new maneuvers and for familiar maneuvers when he's even just a bit rusty. Obviously, some pilots are safe flying below the 1500-foot minimum, a fact recognized by the FAA, which issues altitude waivers to such pilots after they demonstrate their competence. Waivers are issued for various minimum altitudes, starting from the ground. These waivers reflect not only the flying skill but also the judgment of the pilot. Such low altitude pilot waivers can only be exercised where an appropriate airspace waiver exists.

There can be too much of a good thing and more altitude is not always better. Since the pressure of air drops by about 3 percent for each 1000 feet of altitude, the power of a non-supercharged internal combustion engine drops by about the same amount and the climb performance drops even faster. This power loss changes the flying characteristics of the aircraft.

A different problem is found on hazy days, where very high altitudes can cause one to lose sight of the horizon and the visual orientation it gives to the pilot. This condition requires careful handling. If the conditions are such that you cannot reach your safe altitude without a potential loss of references, then it is time to wash the plane, change the oil or engage in some similar ground activity. Federal Aviation Regulations call for a minimum flight visibility of three miles for aerobatic flight. Like the altitude restriction, this is again a minimum value and any condition of less than five miles visibility needs to be handled with care because of orientation problems.

WHO CAN DO AEROBATICS?

There are no airmen certificates that define who can legally do aerobatics and who cannot. This means that the system is self-regulating, and invites abuse from those pilots who figure that they can do aerobatics without training. This type of abuse is often accompanied by a disregard for many of the other legal and common sense rules that we have presented in this chapter. If American aerobatics is to continue to enjoy its freedom from legal interference, then we need to make sure that new pilots are adequately trained before going off on their own. Since there is no aerobatic pilot certificate, there are no certificated aerobatic flight instructors. This means that the prospective student may encounter a wide spectrum of capabilities among the individuals who have hung out their shingles as aerobatic flight instructors. Indeed, there may be some who have done nothing beyond the spins required for the Certified Flight Instructor certificate, so ask some questions before getting started. A good instructor will have plenty of aerobatic experience before he takes on aerobatic students, a fact that can be determined quickly by direct questioning. If he takes offense at detailed questions, then you're obviously talking to the wrong person. As in other activities, experience counts and you should find out if an instructor has had other students and what their experiences were. Finally, a prospective student should expect to see a well-defined program of instruction, indicating adequate planning and preparation.

There is no substitute for aerobatic dual and the interested pilot should seek out an appropriate instructor. The International Aerobatic Club, which we'll discuss in chapter 11, can provide information about instructors and other aerobatic enthusiasts in all parts of the country. The novice aerobat who has only a book as a guide has a poor instructor indeed; however, there will be a point at which the new aerobatic pilot is safe to be on his own. This point is reached when he can do the basic maneuvers well and can recover from muffed maneuvers quickly and correctly. At this point, he can probably attack alone the many variations on the maneuvers that have been mastered. But take this advice with caution. Certainly, when new types of maneuvers are attacked, it should be dual. That this is sound advice is underlined by the case of a super pilot and former national champion who took dual instruction when being introduced to inverted flat spins, maneuvers he had not done earlier. His is an example we should all follow.

Aerobatics can be started very early in a pilot's career, with an introduction before the private license probably advisable to show that stalls and steep bank turns are not excursions to the edge of self-destruction. The recently licensed private pilot should have all of the basic skills for taking on aerobatics, and this is an excellent time to get started. There is a big gap in experience between the private license, obtained at about 40 hours, and the instrument rating at 200 hours and the commercial ticket at 250 hours. After the challenge of the private license, the new pilot often finds when he has flown his family and friends around the local area and tried a few cross-country trips and been weathered-in that there aren't many challenges available to him. Many pilots then stop flying. Any time is a good time to learn aerobatics, but the post-private license is an especially good time.

People do aerobatics for many reasons, but the only good ones come under the term *personal fulfillment,* a fulfillment that can be found privately or publicly. Doing aerobatics well is a challenge some enjoy addressing alone, while others relish the pressure of competition. Some pilots simply want to become safer pilots, a fine goal too. If, however, aerobatics are approached by the desire to attract the attention of others or to demonstrate how fearless one is, then the money is better invested in some "couch" time with another type of licensed professional. The hourly rates are similar and it uses less gas. We have our share of these types too, but the most dramatic change in American aerobatics has been the movement away from stunt flying to a disciplined activity that offers all the challenges a healthy individual can desire.

4
Maneuvers—
Getting Started

THE NUMBER of recognized aerobatic maneuvers is in the thousands, which immediately raises the question of where does one get started? Fortunately, this question becomes simplified when it is recognized that these thousands of maneuvers are composed of combinations of only a relatively few types of maneuvers. These maneuver types should be mastered in their simplest forms, both in execution and understanding, before the compound versions are attacked; otherwise, the poor foundation will show its weakness at some later time and progress will grind to a stop.

Even among the simple forms of the aerobatic maneuvers there is a natural progression that will allow steady advancement. This is the desired result with any learning activity and is done here by addressing the maneuvers in a sequence that presents the new challenges one at a time, mastering them, then building on those skills in the next maneuver. Some types of maneuvers are fundamentally different, for example Loops and

31

Spins, and can be done in parallel to one another. Some types should be introduced later because of the possibility of disorientation; these will be pointed out.

STRAIGHT LINES

What better place is there to start than the beginning and what can be simpler than straight lines? It is necessary to understand how to fly lines because they form a part of every aerobatic maneuver. In fact, national and international rules for competition require that every maneuver begin and end in level flight. Sometimes this can be inverted flight, but the elements are the same as those we'll consider here for upright flight; the differences will be discussed in chapter 6.

The key element in flying straight lines is the distinction between attitude and track. Both are important, and sometimes correct attitude is the desired goal, other times track is relevant.

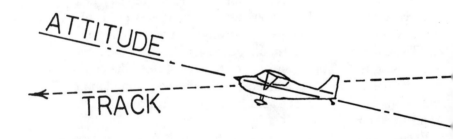

IV-1

Attitude is the direction the airplane is pointed, track is the direction that it is flying. The two directions can be quite different.

Attitude is the orientation of the axis of the aircraft above and below the local level (the horizon on a clear day). Track is the path with respect to the ground that is described by the airplane as it is flying. These are quite different, but nonetheless closely related. How they are related will become clear as we discuss level, climbing and descending lines.

Consider an aircraft in level flight at a constant airspeed. In this case, its track will be constant and level. Its attitude will be constant, but not necessarily level. This is because the air-

INCIDENCE

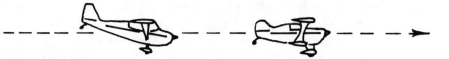

HIGH SPEED FLIGHT(UPRIGHT)

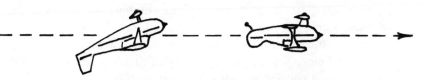

INVERTED FLIGHT(FAST)

IV-2

Incidence describes the angle at which the wings are attached to the airplane. The monoplane shown has large positive incidence while the biplane has little. This makes for highly different attitudes for high speed upright and inverted flight in this monoplane.

plane wings are producing an upward lift that exactly equals the weight of the airplane, and the amount of lift depends both upon the angle of attack of the wings and the airspeed. If the airplane wings are attached with a high angle of incidence, then the angle of attack of the wings would be large even when the attitude of the airplane is level. The same might be true for a highly asymmetric wing that produces large positive lift even at low angles of attack. If our aircraft has symmetric airfoils and zero incidence, then it will have a pronounced positive attitude while producing a level track. On the other hand, our high-incidence or high-lift airplane, which looked level when flying level while upright, will have a nose-high attitude when flying level inverted.

Now consider the more complicated case in which the airplane is flying level but the airspeed is changing. In this case, the attitude will have to change as the airspeed changes in order to maintain the straight line track. The rate of the change depends on many factors such as airfoil design, incidence and rate of acceleration/deceleration, but the basic principle will be the same.

The importance of changing the attitude in order to maintain a constant track is emphasized in climbing and descending lines, where the airspeeds are changing rapidly. Angles of 45° and 60° are the ones most commonly seen in aerobatic maneuvers; and since few airplanes can fly at these angles for long, it means that continuous adjustment of attitude is required. Correct track is the desired goal in all straight aerobatic lines with the exception of vertical lines. In vertical lines (both climbing and diving) the attitude is used for judging quality. Since vertical lines are considered in a later chapter, they won't be discussed further here. (At the time that the present edition of this book is being prepared, the rules have changed to judge all straight lines by attitude, not track. It is not clear that this awkward way of judging will be continued, so I have not altered this discussion or that in Chapter XII.)

Because track is measured with respect to the ground, the wind becomes a factor in flying climbing and descending lines. An airplane climbing on a set track into the wind will need a lower attitude than one climbing on the same track angle but with a tail wind. Similar consideration applies to descending lines.

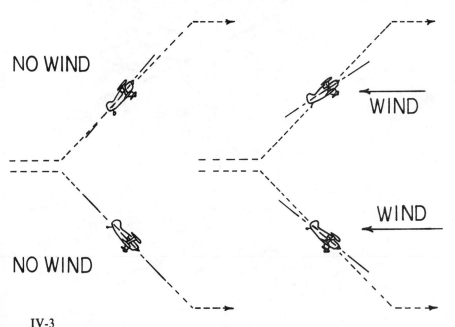

IV-3

Wind makes it necessary to change attitude if an exact 45° flight track is to be flown.

TORQUE

While we are considering lines with varying airspeed, it is appropriate to consider the effects of torque. Since torques produce a turning around the longitudinal (down the middle) axis of the airplane, a drop in a wing can occur (roll). Some

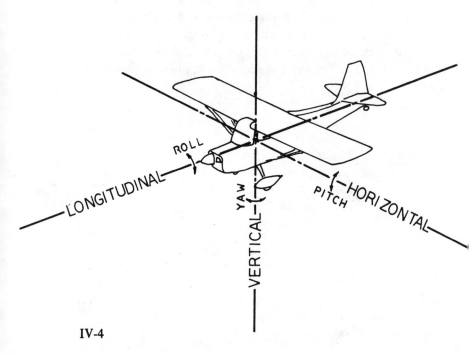

IV-4

The airplane has three axes of orientation and a sense of motion about each.

torques act about the vertical (up through the middle) axis of the airplane, producing a change of heading (yaw). Others work around the horizontal axis (parallel to the wings) and produce attitude changes (pitch). There are four major types of torque: engine torque, slipstream torque, P-factor and precession. We'll treat the first three here and save precession for later.

Engine Torque arises from the natural result of Isaac Newton's law of action and reaction. In this case the engine is turning the propeller clockwise (as viewed by the pilot from behind), which is the action, while the airplane wants to roll counterclockwise, which is the reaction. An airplane is usually rigged so that one wing produces more lift in order to compensate for engine torque, but this will only be correct for one power and airspeed combination; as we change the engine speed in a climb or dive, we'll have to slightly vary the aileron forces in compensation.

Slipstream Torque arises from the corkscrew motion of the air pushed back by the advancing and rotating propeller. More precisely, it is caused by this twisting column of air striking the tail group of the aircraft. The effect is most important when the corkscrew is tight, which is the condition encountered when the engine speed is high and the airspeed low. What happens is that the twisting column of air pushes against the side of the vertical stabilizer and produces a yaw to the left. This is compensated

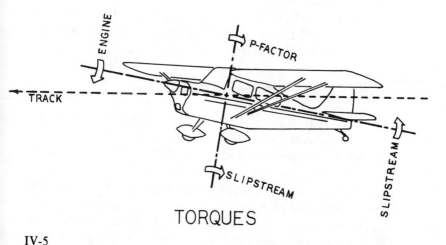

TORQUES

IV-5

Three types of torque compete with one another to disorient the airplane, even in level flight.

for by use of rudder. The twisting column of air also strikes the horizontal stabilizer, from the bottom on the left and from the top on the right, producing a roll to the right, which must be corrected with the ailerons.

P-Factor is often the most important of these three torques. P-factor occurs when the airplane is being flown with its longitudinal axis at an angle to the flight path through the medium of the air. This usually occurs at high angles of attack during climbs. When the angle of attack is positive, the aircraft yaws to its left and when the angle of attack is negative, the aircraft tends to yaw to its right. P-factor is important in higher-power aerobatic airplanes and is noticeable in almost all airplanes during climb.

With all of these torques working on roll and yaw and varying with airspeed and engine speed, it sounds like straight lines are hard to fly. They aren't, but they do require attention to all the controls in the airplane. We must apply such attention if aerobatics are to be truly precision flying. Of course, all of these torques are encountered in other maneuvers as well, with the effects of precession occurring in some cases.

CURVED LINES

Here we will talk only about horizontal curved lines, which means turns. Aerobatic turns employ an angle of bank of at least 60°, meaning that a load factor of at least two G's will be experienced. The roll into and out of the bank should be on the entry and exit headings and the altitude and bank should be constant throughout. Since the airplane is going from one G to two G's at the entry, it is obvious that more lift is needed, hence a need for a higher airspeed or higher angle of attack—or both. Usually one achieves such lift by keeping the speed up and adding more power, which is needed to compensate for the increased drag at the higher angle of attack.

COORDINATED MANEUVERS

There are three closely related maneuvers that are usually introduced early in an aerobatic curriculum: the Wingover, the Chandelle and the Barrel Roll. The reason for their early and sequential introduction is that they all involve use of aileron, rudders and elevators in a familiar, coordinated fashion. Moreover, they do not require rapid changes of orientation, nor do they involve negative G forces (only modest positive G forces). They are graceful, smooth maneuvers that build confidence for the next set of challenges.

In these maneuvers, as in all that we will discuss, the entry speeds given will be those appropriate to an airplane characteristic of those in which this maneuver is first encountered. This means that the numbers for Citabrias will dominate for the early maneuvers, the Decathlon will characterize the intermediate and advanced maneuvers and the two-place Pitts will be used for the most advanced maneuvers. In all cases, the placarded entry speeds should be used for your specific airplane. Entry speeds are always given in Indicated Air Speed, the relevant number in describing the expected response in a maneuver.

THE WINGOVER

The Wingover is a reversing maneuver, in which the airplane changes heading by 180°. The first half involves a coordinated climbing turn and the second half involves a coordinated diving turn, so that the start and finish altitudes are the same. When two Wingovers are executed back to back, with turns in opposite directions, the maneuver is called a Lazy Eight, the name arising from the approximate eight traced by the ground path. The Wingover is shown in figure IV–6; it starts in level flight and then a smooth elevator pull is used to initiate a steep climb, quickly followed by the initiation of a coordinated turn. The

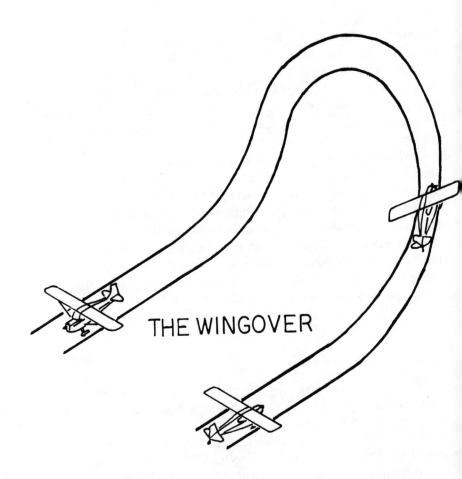

THE WINGOVER

IV-6

The Wingover, described in the text, is usually the student's first introduction to very high angles of bank.

combination of pitch control and rate of turn should be such that when the aircraft has changed heading by 90°, the airspeed is about the stall speed and the angle of bank is about 90°. Good wingovers sometimes have airspeeds at the top that are below the stall speed; this is all right since it is upward momentum that is holding the plane up, not lift from the wings! Once you reach this minimum airspeed point, the nose is allowed to come down as the turn is continued in its same direction. During the second half of the maneuver, the pitch control and rate of turn are combined so that the airplane returns to its original altitude just as the 180° heading is reached. Full power will be used during the first half, to give the most altitude gain and the longest execution time. This means that in order to prevent overspeeding the engine, you will probably need to reduce the power as the airplane builds up airspeed on the descending leg of the maneuver. Even if you use a constant-speed propeller airplane, you'll probably need to monitor the power in order to conclude the maneuver at the entry speed (120 mph in the Citabria). This will allow the immediate entry into a Wingover in the opposite direction, thus completing the Lazy Eight.

Flying the Wingover includes many of the procedures common to all aerobatic maneuvers. First is the need to be clear of other traffic. There is no adequate substitute for the clearing turn and the swivel neck. Next is the utility of good ground references. If you are flying in an area with section lines, start and finish your maneuvers right on a set of these lines. If section lines are not available, use a long straight section of road or railway bed. Finally, Wingovers demonstrate the need to use correct entry speeds.

Entry speeds vary enormously among different maneuvers, and any particular airplane may not be able to reach all entry speeds from full power level flight. In such a case, one needs to dive to pick up the additional airspeed. While performing maneuvers that require a dive for the correct entry speed, it is best to obtain an airspeed a few miles per hour higher than the entry speed, then hold the airplane level until the speed has slowed to the entry speed before initiating the maneuver. Not only will this give the straight line required for the initial part of every aerobatic maneuver, but it will also allow a quick check for wings level and other traffic.

Aircraft with fixed-pitch propellers may have a tendency to overspeed the engine (rpm greater than the red line) during the dive to entry speed. If so, the throttle must be retarded during the approach dive. Of course, the same thing will be true whenever a sustained power-on dive is encountered during the execution of other maneuvers. Exceeding the red line of an engine does produce more power, but you are then operating the engine beyond its design. Engine manufacturers offer no responsibility for performance above the red line and even consider such operation grounds for voiding the engine warranty. The moral of this story is "Don't bust the red line." In unlimited competition, where pilots frequently operate experimental engines, the red line is often just a reference point passed immediately before the first vertical rolling turn, but these pilots are not violating any legal restriction, nor do they expect to reach the normal time between overhauls for that basic engine.

THE CHANDELLE

The Chandelle is a method of reversing heading by 180° while making a maximum increase in altitude (figure IV–7). The entry speed is usually similar to that of the Wingover, as are the maximum G forces (about two to two and a half G's). After establishing level flight, a coordinated turn is begun, immediately followed by the initiation of a steep climb. In this case, the combination of pitch and turn is made so that the airplane reaches the 180° heading exactly as the airspeed reaches slightly above the stall speed, at which time it flies off in level flight on the new heading. Full power should be used as soon as the climb is initiated at a rate to avoid overspeeding the engine.

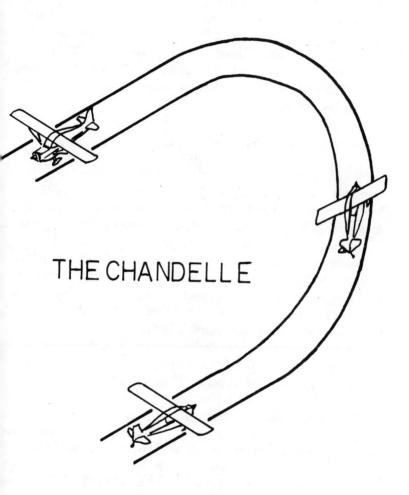

THE CHANDELLE

IV-7

The Chandelle is a coordinated turn-reversing maneuver during which the maximum amount of altitude is gained.

Once in, full power should be left in until after completion of the establishment of level at the end. As in the Wingover, more power gives a longer, more graceful maneuver. The best Chandelles have the maximum pitch angle after 90° of turn and begin decreasing the bank at about this same point. Since the radius of turn decreases with airspeed, the bank angle will be continuously decreasing as the airplane climbs and loses airspeed during the last 90° of turn.

THE BARREL ROLL

Like the preceding maneuvers, the Barrel Roll is fun. Done smoothly and properly, it offers an exhilarating introduction to brief inverted flight and rolling maneuvers. The airplane always seems under highly positive control, there are no side loads and, best of all, the pilot and passenger are still fixed in their seats even when the airplane is inverted! Smooth and confident pilots can execute Barrel Rolls with a glass full of water sitting on top of the instrument panel, without spilling a drop. The Barrel Roll uses many of the skills developed in the Wingover and Chandelle but carries them much farther.

The Barrel Roll is illustrated in figures IV–8 and IV–9. The first figure shows how the maneuver looks from the air, the second figure, from the airplane. The second figure is the more important as it shows what needs to be done. In brief form, what is done is that the aircraft is flown about an imaginary distant point on the horizon, so that the longitudinal axis describes a circle of 20° radius about that point, as seen by the pilot.

The maneuver again begins with level flight and high cruising airspeed (120 mph in the Citabria). A point on the horizon at 20° off heading is selected (either left or right). Your selection is important, as it will be the reference throughout the Barrel Roll. A climbing turn is initiated in the direction of the refer-

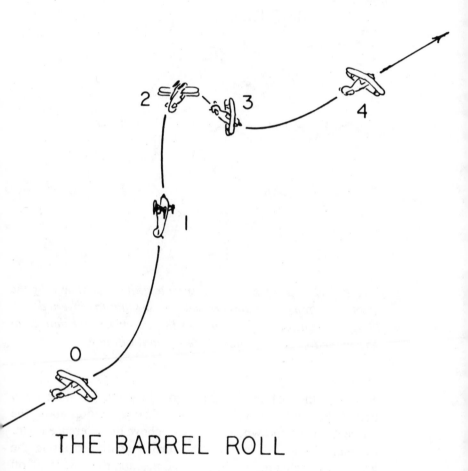

THE BARREL ROLL

IV-8

The Barrel Roll is so named because it involves a flight path about an imaginary cylinder (barrel). The numbered positions correspond to the next figure.

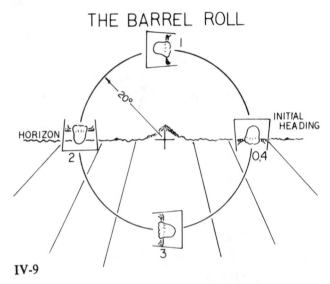

IV-9

The Barrel Roll is flown with respect to attitude as viewed by the pilot. By comparing numbers, you can see that the inverted attitude occurs at the highest point of the maneuver and that all of the maneuver is flown above the original altitude.

ence point in a fashion that the longitudinal axis (the nose if you prefer) describes the first part of a circle of 20° radius about the reference point and when the nose is above the reference point, the bank angle will be 90°. The turn is continued along the imaginary circle until at the inverted position the nose is 40° off the original heading. From then on, the turn about the circle is continued, passing the second 90° bank when the nose is pointed 20° below the reference point, and returning to upright flight on the original heading and altitude.

Comparison of figures IV–8 and IV–9 shows that in actual-

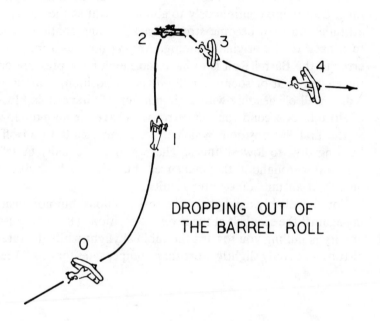

DROPPING OUT OF
THE BARREL ROLL

IV-10

If the nose gets too low at the top of the Barrel Roll, you will probably recover off the original heading and at a much lower altitude and higher airspeed.

ity, the airplane should be climbing through almost all of the first 180° of roll (until inverted flight) and will be diving during the second half. Even though the nose is back on the horizon at the inverted position, this should be the maximum attitude position. The elevator forces will be strong (back) at the beginning, decreasing continuously to about neutral at the inverted attitude and then become strong (back) as one continues the turn back to the original heading. Among novices a frequent error in the Barrel Roll is to have too much back pressure on the elevators at or soon after the inverted position, leading to a dive well off heading with a big buildup of airspeed and loss of altitude. A second common error is to have the nose too low at the first 90° position, which usually then leads to an off-heading dive to low altitudes. The power can usually be left constant throughout the maneuver, but should be reduced quickly if an unplanned dive results.

You'll probably feel light in the seat cushions, but not pushing against the seat belt at the inverted position. This is because gravity is pulling you toward the cabin skylight while the rate-of-turn force only slightly more than compensates for this force.

5
Maneuvers—
The Building
Blocks

In the previous chapter we considered the most basic elements of the precision flying of aerobatics—lines and coordinated maneuvers. The lines will appear in all other maneuvers you will hear about, see, learn or read about. The coordinated maneuvers are basically ends in themselves, except for the control of combinations of forces that they develop. In this chapter we will emphasize the building blocks, those maneuvers that alone, together or in combination form the largest part of aerobatic flying. We'll start with the Loop, develop the Loop in its common combinations with Rolls and finally address the autorotation maneuvers, the Spin and Snap Roll.

THE LOOP

No other maneuver looks so simple, is so simple to do in its most rudimentary form and yet is so difficult to do exactly right. It takes little skill to bring an airplane to entry speed and then

49

pull back until an aerial somersault is performed. It takes a fine touch on elevator, aileron and rudder to perform a Loop that is a thing of beauty. It is important to learn and understand the Loop well because it is the basis of many of the other maneuvers one sees and does.

In an ideal Loop the flight path is a straight line, followed by a perfectly round circle, followed by a second straight line at the same altitude. It is flown by attaining entry speed (140 mph in the Citabria), then initiating a smooth, strong back stick pressure (pitch up), pulling about three to three and a half G's.

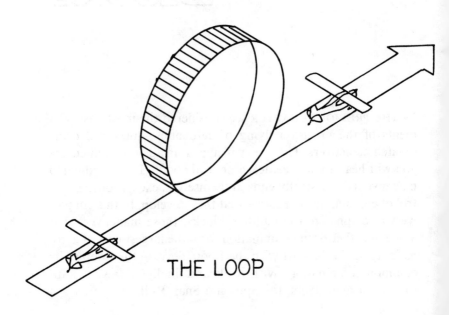

THE LOOP

V-1

The Loop is flown with perfect roundness and the same entry and exit altitudes. The bottom of the flight path is shown by the lined side of the ribbon.

As the airspeed diminishes and the nose passes about 45° beyond the vertical, the back pressure is lessened and the airplane literally floats across the top. Once you have passed the inverted position and the nose has started down, the airspeed increases rapidly and strong back pressure is again necessary if the Loop is to be round and the entry altitude is to be matched at the bottom. The most common error in Loops is the inaccurate balance of airspeed, position and elevator control. This results in Loops that look like script l's or e's, or like printed D's, or even the printer's delete symbol, as shown in figure V–2. Full power should be used at least until you pass the inverted position, when power can be retarded. Use of power on the way down depends on the exit speed desired.

Heading control must be maintained throughout the Loop. Mastery of heading control starts even before the initial pull.

THE LOOP

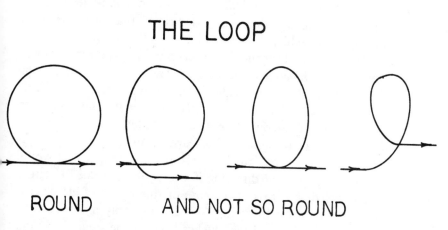

ROUND   AND NOT SO ROUND

V-2

A perfect Loop is rarely encountered. If the pilot uses an inappropriate variation of back elevator pressure, almost any closed figure can result. These are some of the most common.

You can best judge heading by first looking to see if the wings are level, then returning your gaze straight forward just as the pull is initiated. As the horizon disappears beneath the rising nose, your gaze can be turned sideways so that passage through the vertical can be judged. As the inverted (180° point) is approached, the horizon again comes into view ahead and you can look forward throughout the rest of the trip around.

If you use only elevator control at the beginning of the Loop, you will be in for a surprise when reaching the inverted position, for the airplane will undoubtedly be well off the desired heading and one wing will probably be down. This is because the turning forces of engine, slipstream and P-factor torque have all been acting on the airplane. All of these torques act in constantly varying amounts to roll the airplane wing down and to take it off heading. Such forces require continuous attention to attitude and correction. Experience will show how much correction is needed and when. It is, of course, better to apply these corrections as they are needed rather than after they have become noticeable.

One additional turning force becomes important in the Loop and that is *Propeller Gyroscopic Precession Torque,* precession for short. [Since this torque is important for understanding Loops, as well as later maneuvers, we'll interrupt our discussion to explain precession.] Many of us studied the workings of gyroscopic instruments when learning instrument flight. At that time we learned that an axis of a spinning wheel would change in a peculiar direction if a force were applied to either the wheel or the axis. The sense of this result of action and reaction is shown in figure V–3. If you apply a force to the spinning wheel, the wheel pushes back in the same direction, but 90° ahead. The same process occurs in the airplane because the spinning propeller functions as a rotating wheel. As the airplane is pitched up upon entry to a Loop, it is as if a forward force were applied at the bottom of the propeller disk. The

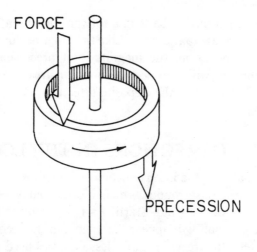

V-3

A spinning disk shows the effect of gyroscopic precession. If a force is applied at one point of the disk, the disk reacts by applying a similar force (precession) 90° ahead.

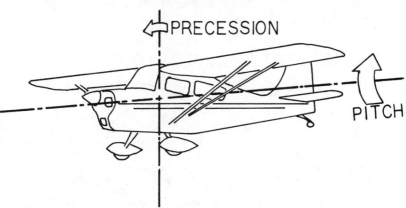

V-4

As the airplane is pitched nose up, the spinning disk of the propeller acts as if it is being pushed forward on the bottom. The resulting precession force acts to yaw the airplane to the right.

propeller then pushes back in a forward direction, making the nose tend to yaw to the right. Like the other perturbing torques acting on the Loop, the magnitude of precession will vary. Sometimes it will compensate for slipstream and P-factor torque, which act in the opposite direction and at other times it will not.

WIND CORRECTIONS IN THE LOOP

The quality of the Loop depends on how round it looks when viewed from the ground, which means that we must apply corrections for the wind. Starting a Loop into the wind means that the first half will appear flattened and the second half will look bulged (figure V-5). Thus, less G forces need to be pulled when you are headed into the wind, during the first and last quarters of the Loop, and more G's on the top half. Since the natural tendency seems to be to pinch the top halves of Loops, especially the third quarter, it's usually easier to start Loops into the wind. If the Loop is entered with a tail wind, then the corrections would be opposite.

EFFECT OF WIND ON LOOPS

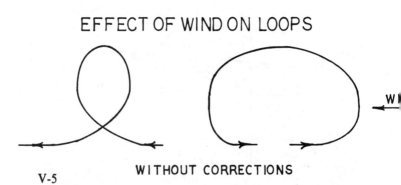

V-5

WITHOUT CORRECTIONS

The perfect Loop must compensate for the effects of wind. There will be headwind and tailwind components throughout the Loop. If corrections are not applied, these figures will result.

G FORCES IN THE LOOP

Since the G forces in the Loop are the highest encountered thus far, this is a good place to consider the origin of these forces and how to control them. In chapter 2, we explained that G forces resulted from the momentum of an airplane, which wants to carry it straight forward. In a change of pitch or direction, we move at an angle. This gives rise to the physicist's "imaginary" force, centrifugal force, which seems anything but imaginary when you're experiencing it. Scientists call it an imaginary force because nothing is actually pushing you out; it's your momentum that makes you feel that way. Centrifugal force can be expressed as pounds, but it is more convenient to use the ratio to the ordinary weight, which is G force. This means that if you ordinarily weigh 170 pounds, under five G's you'd weigh 850 pounds (you'd better be in a well-padded seat when you do!).

The amount of the G force depends upon your speed and the radius of the turn about the middle of the Loop. For a constant radius, the G force goes up as the speed is squared (multiplied by itself). For a constant speed, the G force goes down as the radius increases. (For the mathematically inclined, this means that the G force varies as speed^2 divided by radius.)

At the beginning of a Loop (the first portion level flight), we experience the one G of gravity, but as the nose is pitched up, the load increases rapidly. Figure V-6 shows a Loop in which five G's are pulled at entry. Five G's are too much for an ordinary Loop, but the example provides an easy explanation. One G is still there because of gravity and the other four result from centrifugal force. As the airplane climbs it loses speed.

If the Loop is truly round and if the airspeed drops to one-half the entry speed at the top, then the centrifugal force at the top is still pushing you into your seat and is now only one G. Likewise, gravity is still one G but is pulling you out of your

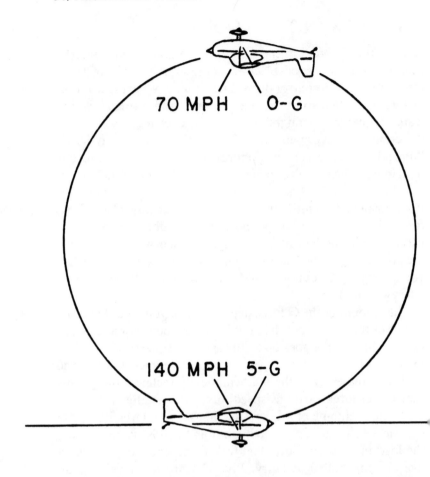

70 MPH 0-G

140 MPH 5-G

G FORCES IN THE LOOP

V-6

At the bottom of a Loop, the centrifugal force is added to gravity to produce a high G load. At the top of the Loop the centrifugal force is smaller and in the opposite direction to gravity. The right combination of speeds and entry G can produce weightlessness on top.

seat. The two forces would exactly balance and you would float as weightless as any astronaut at the top of your Loop! Ordinary Loops will not have exactly this combination of speeds and entry G forces, but the type and direction of the forces will be the same.

THE CUBAN EIGHT

There are many types of rolling maneuvers and they will be presented here in a natural order of progression. We start with the maneuver in which it is easy to introduce the partial Roll. The name *Cuban Eight* has its origin in obscure flying lore, although the most popular story attributes both the name and the maneuver to a gringo who developed the new maneuver in Cuba. The Cuban Eight is five-eighths of a Loop followed by a straight line with a one-half Slow Roll in the middle, with a recovery to level. In its complete form, this sequence is then repeated, thereby forming a figure eight when viewed from the side. We'll discuss it as a full figure, although this form is normally used only in demonstration and recreational flying.

Figure V-7 illustrates the Cuban Eight. You'll see that this is our first introduction to sustained inverted flight and the roll, each in a simplified form. The first part, the five-eighths Loop, is flown exactly as in the round Loop, perhaps with a little more entry speed (145 mph in the Citabria), except that as the nose reaches 45° below the horizon, forward stick is applied, pinning the nose and flying a brief accelerating inverted line. In an aircraft without an inverted fuel system, the engine will stop firing, but since the aircraft is accelerating, the propeller will usually continue windmilling and the engine will begin firing on its own after the later recovery to upright flight. The airplane is rolled upright on the 45° down line by application of full aileron. In order to keep the nose from dropping and to prevent the airplane from dropping below the track established before

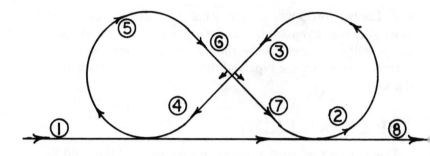

V-7 THE CUBAN EIGHT

The Cuban Eight is a combination of partial Loops, 45° dives and Half Rolls. This complex maneuver is best followed by observing the arrows and position numbers. The positions of the Half Rolls are shown by the short barbs.

the roll began, top rudder will be needed as you pass the knife-edge position. In this case, the rudder used will be in the same direction as the aileron, that is, right rudder with right aileron and vice versa. Most airplanes roll faster to the left, and this is the most common way of doing the half roll.

Top rudder use is necessary to conteract the loss of lift that occurs as the wings roll from the horizontal. When the airplane begins its 45° diving line, the wings have a small negative angle of attack that keeps the airplane flying. The increasing tilt of the wings during the roll means progressively less upward lift is available. At the plane's knife-edge position, the wings aren't producing any upward lift. The lift must then come from the fuselage, acting as an airfoil, and the top rudder puts in the necessary positive angle of attack. This means that the rudder deflection will be zero at the start, maximum at 90° of roll and zero again at upright. Of course, such use of rudder also works to overcome the effects of adverse yaw—caused by the downward deflected ailerons exerting greater drag. In this case, adverse yaw also tends to pull the nose down.

After the airplane has completed its Half Roll, the 45°

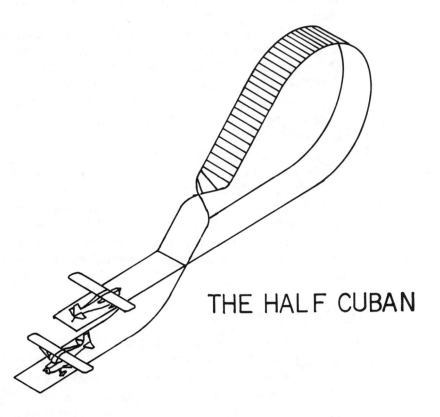

V-8

The Half Cuban is a reversing maneuver with careful attention paid to roundness of the Five-Eighths Loop and equal length line segments before and after the Half Roll.

down line should be continued for the same distance as the line before the roll. Since the speed is now much higher, the time spent on this leg will be much shorter. You should allow the speed to build up so that you reach the original entry speed as you have leveled out and immediately pull for the start of the second half of the figure eight.

The prettiest Cuban Eights have circles of the same radius, exact heights at the two tops and bottoms and perfectly matched, intersecting 45° lines, with the two Half Rolls centered on the same spot. Such precision is a tall order in any circumstance and becomes a real challenge if there is a wind. All of the corrections cited earlier for flying straight lines and round Loops with a wind apply here, because one half will have a head wind and the other half will have a tail wind.

When the Half Cuban is flown as a reversing maneuver (figure V-8), the procedures are all the same as above, except that the recovery is made to level flight after the first down line. In this case, the final altitude does not have to be the same as entry altitude, which gives the pilot more opportunity to set good lines and to obtain a different entry speed for the next maneuver.

THE IMMELMANN

Close cousin to the Half Cuban is the Immelmann, which is simply a Half Loop followed by a Half Roll. The name for this maneuver is, like the Chandelle, historical, going back to World War I. However, like many historical allusions, the original tie to the German Ace Max Immelmann is not all that firm. It isn't established that he ever did this maneuver in his dogfighting days, but the name is there nevertheless.

A higher entry speed than in the Loop is needed for the Immelmann (145 mph in the Citabria) and a tighter radius (about three and a half G's). This gives a higher airspeed at the

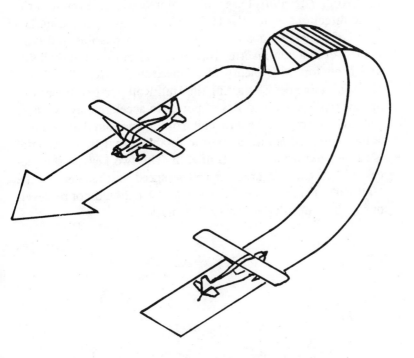

THE IMMELMANN

V-9

The Immelmann is a Half Loop immediately followed by a Half Roll. Since the rolling motion starts at very low airspeed, it is more difficult than the Half Cuban.

top of the Half Loop. Higher airspeed is needed because the plane not only needs flying speed to hold itself up at this slowest point but also requires some extra speed for performing the Half Roll. The control use will be more extreme, even if in the same directions as for the Half Cuban, because the rising airspeed of the Half Cuban is not present. It is possible to do this maneuver in a non-inverted fuel system aircraft, but only if you arrive on top with plenty of airspeed and barely "kiss" the horizontal line before starting the Half Roll portion. Even with an inverted system and lots of power to accelerate away, there should be no more than a touching of the horizontal line on top. What is needed is just enough to establish that the horizontal is recognized prior to the Half Roll. The two keys to the successful Immelmann are sufficient airspeed and mastery of the Half Roll at slow airspeed. This maneuver should not be developed, then, until after the Roll is mastered.

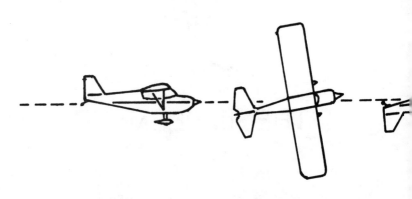

THE SLOW ROLL

THE ROLL

Like the Loop, the Roll is one of the basic elements found in many aerobatic maneuvers. It is important to understand it fully. It looks easy, and when mastered it is, but there are enough subtleties to be a challenge to learn and execute well. Since aileron, rudder and elevator controls are all used and in rapid succession, at first you will feel as though you've been asked to rub your head, pat your stomach and polka at the same time. Fortunately, this feeling quickly passes.

The Roll (more precisely, the Slow Roll) is a complete rotation of the airplane about its longitudinal axis, maintaining constant altitude, heading and rate of rotation throughout (figure V-10). The requirements seem simple; let's see what it takes to fly it.

As remarked in chapter 2, a given aircraft rolls faster at

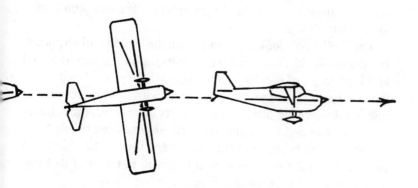

V-10

The Roll (or Slow Roll) is done at constant altitude and rate of roll. The attitude of the aircraft must be adjusted continuously to adjust for varying lift from the wings and the fuselage.

higher speeds, up to the point that control pressures become too high and higher level aerodynamic effects begin to enter. Since the airplane will be flying inefficiently while nonlevel, it will tend to slow down during the Roll unless plenty of power is available. These considerations give a range of possible entry speeds, but in an aircraft like the Citabria, 120 mph gives good performance. Following the establishing of a level flight track, full aileron is smoothly but quickly applied, immediately followed by a slight nose-up pitch and addition of opposite rudder to compensate for loss of upward lift. After 90° of rotation, strong opposite (top) rudder will be needed to prevent loss of altitude and some forward pitch will be needed to keep on heading. By the time the inverted position is being passed, the nose will need to be high enough (push forward) to keep the airplane from settling and rudder pressure will have been relaxed. The second half of the Roll follows in the same way, except now the top rudder at the second knife-edge position will be in the same sense as the aileron. It all happens fast, but if you've been doing Half Cubans before, adding the first half of the Roll, in order to make the complete maneuver won't seem as difficult.

The Roll won't look or sound quite the same in all airplanes. In an airplane like the Citabria, with its high-lift wings attached at a high angle of incidence, the nose will be pushed quite high when passing inverted, as compared with symmetric airfoil, low-incidence wing planes like the Pitts. Moreover, the roll rate will be slower and the engine will probably hesitate briefly from fuel starvation in the light trainers. Nevertheless, the quality of the maneuver depends on how it is flown, in terms of its basic elements and not on nose attitude or sound level.

Misjudged use of rudder and elevator can produce heading changes and altitude fluctuations that normally are only annoying. In the early stages of learning the maneuver, misuse of elevator control at the inverted position can produce a poten-

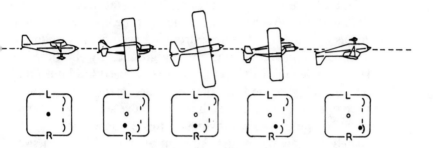

FIRST HALF-SLOW ROLL, VIEWED FROM ABOVE.

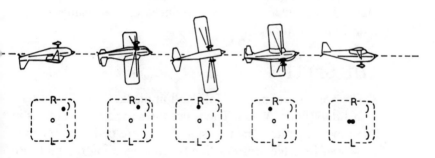

SECOND HALF—SLOW ROLL, VIEWED FROM BELOW.

V-11

A right Roll is shown step by step. The control positions are depicted below the aircraft. The filled circles show the stick position and the semicircles represent the rudders. The open circle and dashes show the neutral positions.

tially dangerous situation. Many students don't take out the initial back pressure that was put in at the start and find themselves with the nose below the horizon at the inverted position. This usually leads to the nose dropping even further, followed by the airplane accelerating for the ground. By the time the plane is pulled back to level flight, the airspeed has built up to uncomfortably beyond the recommended maneuvering speed, the engine has passed the red line and you've set a new personal record for pulling G's. Obviously, this sequence needs to be avoided, the key being just the right amount of forward stick pressure at the inverted position. If you do get into this position, arrest the drop of the nose with forward pressure and roll to upright as fast as possible. If you've discovered the situation too late, turn the power off, pull just enough to keep the speed from building up too much and apply the blackout precautions we will discuss in chapter 8. After recovery from such an unplanned maneuver, you'll be convinced of the wisdom of altitude as life insurance.

THE SPLIT S

The Split S is simply a Half Roll immediately followed by a Half Loop (figure V-12). The procedures are all the same as in these two separate maneuvers, and they are tied together by a very brief inverted straight line before beginning the pull into the Half Loop. This maneuver is usually introduced later than the Roll since the Half Roll must be done at a very low speed (80 mph in the Citabria); otherwise, the speed will be too high at the bottom of the Half Loop. Even a familiar amount of G forces may cause some vision graying because of the brief period of inverted flight that precedes the high G loads. In addition to the physiological controls that can be applied, one can stay out of trouble by retarding power as the nose starts down while inverted.

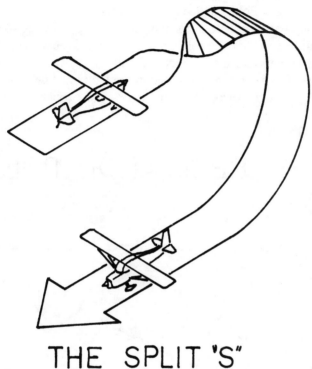

THE SPLIT 'S'

V-12

The Split S is the opposite of the Immelmann. The usual first impressions from the Split S are how much altitude is lost and how the G load can cause you to gray out or black out.

HESITATION ROLLS

A natural variation on the Roll is the hesitation roll. In this maneuver the aircraft is stopped momentarily at a predetermined number of positions as it rolls. The most common hesitation roll is the Four Point Roll, in which the airplane stops rotation every 90°. Of course, there are many others: Three Point, Eight Point, Sixteen Point and so on.

The challenge here is to make sure the pauses are of equal duration and that the roll rate is the same for each leg. These requirements are made more difficult by the fact that all the control force combinations used in the Roll must be applied for a long enough period that any errors will probably show up.

HESITATION ROLLS

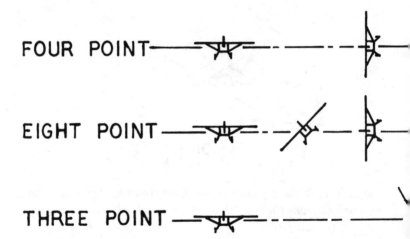

FOUR POINT

EIGHT POINT

THREE POINT

Since the aircraft will be held inverted for brief periods, a non-inverted systems aircraft will have to bring extra airspeed to the entry. Without the extra airspeed, the slowing down of the airplane after the engine stops will cause the pilot to rush the last points. Since most aircraft without inverted fuel systems also lack inverted oil supplies, performing sustained inverted flight produces engine abuse and an oily aircraft when you land.

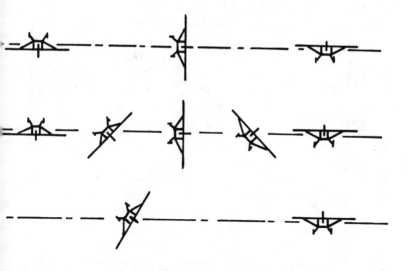

V-13

There are many variations on the Hesitation Rolls, with three of them displayed here as viewed from the rear. Each point of hesitation is shown.

AUTOROTATION

The pilot is accustomed to operating aircraft in equilibrium conditions, such as level flight, steady climbs and glides, but there are additional flight conditions that are equally stable but not usually encountered. These conditions are called autorotation and are encountered in Spins and Snap Rolls. Unfortunately, Spins are no longer encountered in most pilot training, with the predictable resulting number of accidents.

Autorotation can be understood easily by examination of figure V-14, in which we show the coefficient of lift plotted against the angle of attack of a wing. The coefficient of lift gives

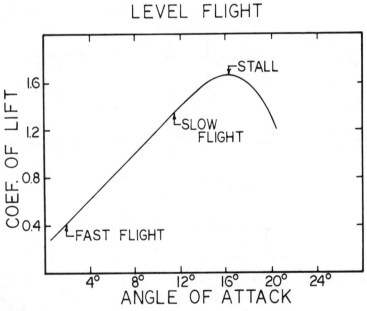

V-14
The coefficient of lift increases with larger angle of attack until the point of stall is reached.

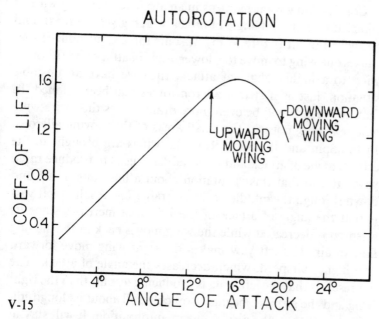

V-15

If the wings are yawed while at the point of stall, the rearward moving wing will enter a deeper stall and the forward will unstall. The stalled wing drops while the other rises, a stable condition known as autorotation.

a measure of how much lift a wing produces per square foot of surface at a fixed speed. In high speed flight, in which there is a high flow of air across the wing, only a low coefficient of lift is needed to sustain level flight and hence a small angle of attack is used. When the airplane is flown slower, there is less flow of air, a larger coefficient of lift is needed and a higher angle of attack is used. This trend is continued as an airplane slows until the maximum coefficient of lift position is reached. If the airplane is slowed any further (the nose raised any more), the lift decreases and the wings stall.

Consider now what happens in an airplane operating with its wings at that critical angle of attack which gives the maximum coefficient of lift (figure V-15). If some force is introduced that causes one wing to move to a lower angle of attack and the other wing to a higher angle of attack, then we have an unstable situation, just as if strong aileron forces had been applied. In fact, the results will be even more dramatic, as the entire wing will be acting, not just the small areas of the moving ailerons. In the Spin and the Snap Roll, the wings are brought to the critical angle of attack and then rudder is used to produce rapid yaw. (Recall that this is rotation about a line running up and down through the middle of the aircraft.) The result of left yaw is that the angle of attack of the left wing increases since its airspeed is decreased while the wing moves back in the moving flow of air. The left yaw makes the right wing move forward at a higher airspeed, which decreases the angle of attack. The net result is that the left wing is producing less lift than the right wing and the airplane begins to quickly roll about its longitudinal axis—that is, the airplane is in autorotation. It will stay in autorotation until the uneven angle-of-attack condition of the wings is altered.

THE SPIN

The most common form of autorotation maneuver is the Spin. In this case, the airplane is at the slowest possible airspeed as the wings are brought to the critical angle of attack and the autorotation is introduced by use of rudder. The forward speed immediately drops and the airplane rapidly transitions to a vertical flight path, a condition that continues until the appropriate recovery techniques are applied. It is this basic stability of the Spin that makes it dangerous to the undertrained pilot, who cannot recognize a Spin or who is so confused by his first (accidental) encounter that he doesn't recover correctly. Once

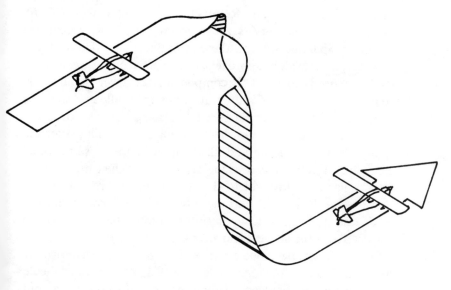

V-16 # THE SPIN

The Spin is entered from level flight, with the airplane slowed to the stall point as autorotation is started. Recovery is followed by a vertical dive and recovery to high-speed level flight.

the pilot is trained, he will find the Spin a docile maneuver, no more demanding than the recovery on heading from a steep turn.

As elsewhere in this book, we'll describe the Spin as an aerobatic maneuver, with certain procedures differing from those involved with studying the Spin as a safety aid. Likewise, the recovery technique that produces minimum altitude loss may differ among airplane types. There is no substitute for dual instruction in Spins.

The aerobatic or precision Spin has a succession of components: Level Flight, Entry, Autorotation, Stop on Heading,

Vertical Down Line and Return to Level Flight (figure V-16). All of these components are necessary. Let's fly through a one-turn Spin and see how these components are tied together. The airplane usually approaches the Spin from a higher than stall airspeed, so the first component, the level flight track, requires that you smoothly reduce power to idle and increase the angle of attack as the airspeed decreases. The basics of flying a level track are important here, for many beginning aerobatic pilots drift off heading and allow the airplane to settle while they are thinking ahead to the Spin entry. When the angle of attack has been brought to the stall point, where both wings have begun to lose lift and the nose begins to drop, rapid full rudder is applied, inducing the autorotation. The nose will drop to just above the vertical and after the first quarter turn the rate of rotation will be about constant. Full back stick will usually be needed to hold the high angles of attack. Anticipating ahead, in order to come out on heading, you should keep in the full rudder and back stick force until you want the rotation to stop. Opposite rudder is applied, to break the autorotation, and then the nose is pitched forward with the elevator in order to break the stall. Usually one will have to continue the forward motion of the nose in order to reach the vertical dive attitude (not track) that is necessary in the aerobatic Spin.

During the autorotation the airspeed will remain low but as the stalled condition of the wings is ended and the nose comes down, the airspeed will begin to rise rapidly. This means that the stopping of autorotation, breaking of the stall and bringing the airplane to a vertical attitude all need to be one smooth, rapid and continuous activity, otherwise unnecessary altitude loss will result. After the vertical attitude is established, a smooth pull is used to recover level flight. The exit speed and total altitude lost in the Spin depends critically on how tight you pull to level flight and how quickly power is brought back in. It also reflects how long the vertical attitude is held. If power is added just as the vertical attitude is reached and that attitude is held only long enough to establish that you have done this part correctly, then minimum altitude loss and high exit speed can be combined. The Citabria will use up about 800 feet of altitude in an aerobatic Spin.

Doing multiple or fractional Spins is largely just a matter of timing. Some aircraft do change their spin characteristics at higher numbers of turns, rotating faster or slower, with the nose coming up or going down. If you want to experiment with higher numbers of turns, it is wise to get lots of extra altitude, for the plane may not recover as quickly as you expect.

Depending upon the rigging, fuel distribution, propeller size, idle speed and many other factors, airplanes will usually have slightly different spin characteristics in left and right rotation. The best thing is to see what the characteristics of both are, because later you may want to do fractions of turns to use the Spin to change directions.

THE SNAP ROLL

The Snap Roll is a level flight roll in which the ailerons are not necessary. Such a statement should not be surprising to the reader who understands the earlier section on autorotation. Like the Spin, the Snap Roll uses autorotation to roll the airplane, but here the entry speeds are high enough that the flight path remains horizontal. It is often said that the Snap Roll is simply a horizontal spin. More accurately, the Snap Roll is simply horizontal autorotation.

The Snap Roll is entered from level flight at speeds well above stall but below cruise (85 mph in the Citabria). At the correct entry speed the nose is abruptly pitched up so that the wings reach the critical angle of attack and rapid, full rudder is applied to "induce" the autorotation. Power is needed, usually about 50 to 75 percent. This means that the autorotation part is approached from accelerating airspeed or power is added as the snap is begun. The stick-back, full-rudder position is held until just before the wings-level position is reached, when the recovery is initiated. Like the Spin, the rotation is stopped with opposite rudder and then the nose is pitched down to break the stall.

You'll be impressed with the high rate of the autorotation, which is much higher than in the Roll. The other strong impression is from the abrupt high G forces (three to four) that are experienced as the nose is pitched up. It is often said that one pulls the high G's to enter the Snap Roll, but they are actually only a side result of the rapid pitch change at moderate speed. Nevertheless, if you don't pull fast enough to get the G's, you won't get the high angle of attack and airspeed combination necessary for horizontal autorotation.

Because the airplane is in a high drag configuration during the autorotation, the airplane will rapidly decelerate during the Snap Roll, the amount depending on whether or not the stick is kept fully aft all of the way around and on how much power is being used. If the rudder and elevator forces are kept in, the autorotation will continue until the forward speed bleeds off and your Snap Roll decays into a Spin. The first step in the recovery from this circumstance is to reduce power, since the airplane may have entered a flat spin.

The Snap Roll characteristics of a plane differ noticeably when doing them to the left and right. Sometimes Snap Rolls to the left will be faster, since one is moving against the propeller rotation, but the airspeed decreases more and the nose attitude is higher. This characteristic is more pronounced when using higher powers. This is due to the gyroscopic forces of precession of the propeller that we first considered when studying Loops (figure V-17). In the case of a left Snap Roll, the rapid left yaw causes the nose to pitch up, increasing the drag and slowing the autorotation. In the right Snap Roll the nose wants to pitch down to a lower drag, increasing the rate of autorotation (as long as the stick forces are still back).

Probably because of its combination of G loads, rapid rotation and lack of references, the Snap Roll unsettles the stomach of the beginning aerobatic flyer faster than any other basic maneuver. It is best approached after a certain feel for the saddle has been developed and even then only in brief segments at the start.

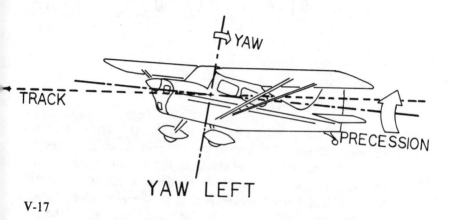

V-17

The rapid yawing motion of the left Snap Roll will cause a precession force that raises the aircraft nose.

6

Maneuvers— Straight Up and Outside

WE HAVE CONSIDERED first those basic maneuvers that make up most of the aerobatic flying done in America. They are within the capability of all aerobatic aircraft and even low-time aerobatic pilots. Now we'll take on the challenge of aerobatics that requires both special systems in the aircraft and more experience and skill on the part of the pilot. Some of the maneuvers are easy but can get you into trouble if done improperly; these have been put here to underline the need for caution. The maneuvers considered here all require sustained vertical flight, sustained inverted flight or negative G forces in their normal execution.

EQUIPMENT

The equipment requirement for these maneuvers is more demanding than that encountered so far. I am speaking not so much of aircraft strength but of fuel and oil systems. In order to continue running in all flight attitudes, an aircraft needs a continuous flow of fuel to the engine, and while it is running it needs continuous lubrication. It is appropriate to digress here on the equipment requirements before considering the maneuvers that impose the demands.

Fuel flow to the engine requires two things: continuous feed from the fuel tank and continuous operation of the carburetor. Feed from the fuel tank is usually guaranteed by one of two approaches, a flop tube or a header tank. The flop tube arrangement (figure VI-1) uses a flexible weighted tube to draw fuel from the tank. The weight pulls the pickup orifice in the same direction that the G forces are pulling the fuel, guaranteeing a steady flow until the fuel is depleted. The header tank approach (figure VI-2) contains no moving parts, but does not allow indefinitely long operation in negative G's. In this arrangement the fuel flows from the main tank into a small (header) tank during positive G loads, which is most of the time for the majority of flights. The fuel is then continuously drawn from the middle of the header tank. Since the header tank does not refill during negative G's, fuel starvation can occur after three to ten minutes, depending on the particular design. Most systems are set up so that the header tank will refill in only a fraction of the fuel starvation time, so alternating positive and negative G flight can continue indefinitely. Most light aircraft engines employ float type carburetors, which will shut off fuel flow to the engine when flying negative G's. The fully aerobatic aircraft usually uses a pressure-diaphragm carburetor or employs a fuel injector system.

An aircraft engine keeps running because of all those thin films of oil that separate the moving metal parts. The engine will self-destruct if run more than a few minutes without oil and will need premature overhaul if frequently run without oil, even if only for brief periods. There are several commercial units available to provide oil to the engine's oil pump, even during

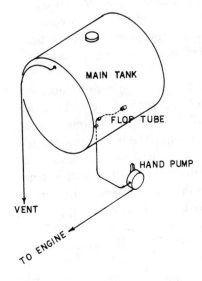

VI-1

The Flop Tube arrangement for inverted fuel supply is lightweight in itself, but requires that several extra gallons of fuel be carried.

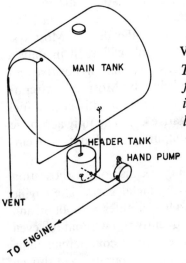

VI-2

The Header Tank arrangement for inverted fuel supply is heavier in itself, but has no moving parts and less fuel is necessary for guaranteed continuous flow. It is not useful for continuous inverted flight, however.

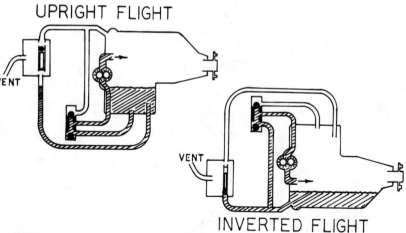

UPRIGHT FLIGHT

VENT

INVERTED FLIGHT

VENT

VI-3

Oil supply and venting of crankcase gases occur through a series of lines and check valves in this system. The check valves prevent air from being mixed with the oil or oil being pushed out the vent line. (After a figure by Christen Industries)

negative G's. The technique used is shown in figure VI-3. The G-force-driven balls in the check valve select whether oil is drawn from the top or bottom of the engine and the oil separator allows the blow-by gases of the crankcase to escape overboard.

VERTICAL LINES

As pointed out earlier, vertical lines are judged on attitude rather than track. The reason for this becomes clear when you consider the problems that would be presented in a wind if track were the criterion. Since the airspeed is changing rapidly and can be lower than the wind speed, flying vertical lines by track

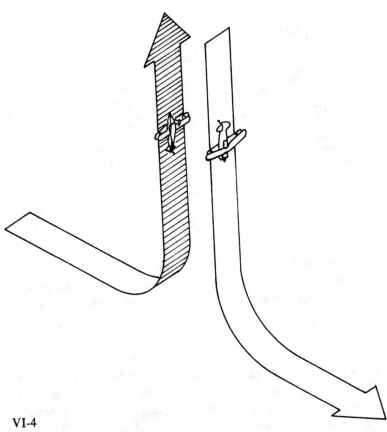

VI-4

Vertical lines are flown with reference to attitude and are always preceded or followed by level flight.

would place the airplane in extreme attitudes on the top. Often such extreme attitudes would prevent execution of the next maneuver or part of a maneuver.

The altitude gained in a climbing vertical line (figure VI-4) depends upon entry speed, entry technique and aircraft performance. Entry speed is important because it gives the airplane high kinetic energy that is only slowly overcome by gravity as the airplane is pointed up. Entry technique is important because the Quarter Loop that marks the transition from level flight to vertical flight is what determines the amount of speed that is left for the vertical line itself. Usually the Quarter Loop will be of smaller radius (tighter) than that of the Loop and Half Loop and will be entered at a higher airspeed. This means that a higher G load will be encountered, usually about five G's. Tighter and faster aren't necessarily better, for one is at the edge of the point at which G load physiological effects begin to become critical. Moreover, when very high G loads are pulled, the wings are operating at high drag and low efficiency. Trial and error will show the best speed and G load for a particular airplane. Once the Quarter Loop is completed and the vertical attitude is assumed, the length of the vertical line depends on the remaining airspeed and the thrust delivered by the engine. This is the point at which the power loading of the airplane makes a big difference. Fortunately for the low-budget pilot the length of the vertical line is not a measure of the quality of a maneuver; it simply limits your ability to add Rolls, Snaps and other exotic features.

The diving vertical line is entered from low airspeeds, so that the principal consideration, after establishing the vertical attitude, is how long the line should be held and how tight the Quarter Loop at the bottom should be. Like the vertical line and Quarter Loop recovery at the end of a Spin, less altitude is lost if power is added during the recovery while still vertical.

Since the airspeed and power are varying rapidly in the vertical lines, they will require close attention to the torque effects that will cause the airplane to roll or yaw.

So far, we have considered only the bottoms and middles of vertical lines, for there are a wide variety of ways of getting out of the vertical up line, which obviously cannot go on forever, transitioning from vertical to level flight (and vice versa) and transitioning from vertical up to vertical down. Now we'll address what goes on at the top.

TRANSITIONING TO THE HORIZONTAL

The vertical climb can be topped off in level flight (figure VI-5) if a fine touch and accurate timing are used. We'll take the example of transitioning to inverted level flight, but the transition can be to either inverted or upright and the differences in technique are rather obvious. The transition, which begins with a backward pull on the stick, must be started with ample airspeed as the airspeed will continue to drop. Simply stated, one can say to pull the nose over until a level flight track is assumed, but there is much more to the maneuver. Too abrupt an application can put the airplane into a level flight attitude but without flying speed. Since the airplane will be far behind on the power curve, it will settle badly before flying speed is reached. Settling will occur even with the full power setting that has been in use since first pulling for the vertical line.

The correct touch is to play the backward force so that the deceleration of gravity is compensated by the horizontal acceleration of the engine. Here one can use centrifugal force to good advantage. Although gravity will always be pulling the airplane down with a force of one G, a component of the outward centrifugal force of this Quarter Loop will be upward and the airplane will effectively weigh less than it did on the ground. This means that less lift will be required from the wings and the airplane can fly perfectly well at below the normal stall speed! This is impressive to watch and even more fun to do. No aerodynamic laws are violated; we just stretch their realm of application. Throughout the transition to the level, the torque factors will all be acting to cause a wing to drop or a heading to change.

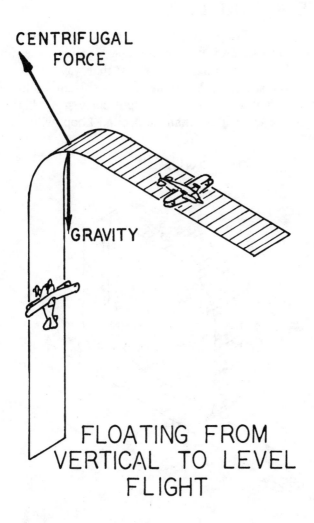

FLOATING FROM VERTICAL TO LEVEL FLIGHT

VI-5

The transition from upward vertical flight to level flight can actually involve flying the airplane slower than the stall speed. This is because the centrifugal force partially compensates for gravity.

THE SQUARE LOOP

The Square Loop ties together the lines and Quarter Loops we have just been discussing into one graceful maneuver. The Square Loop is intended to look just that way (figure VI-6)—that is, four straight sides connected by constant radius Quarter Loops. It is flown with a level flight entry speed higher (145 mph in the Decathlon) than the Round Loop, with the initial

THE SQUARE LOOP

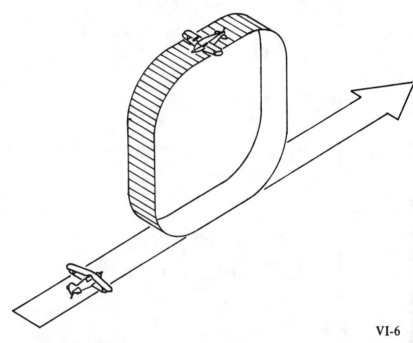

VI-6

The ideal Square Loop has four straight sides of constant length connected by round corners of the same radius. As in executing a round Loop, it is easy to fly, but difficult to fly a perfect one.

pull for the vertical line at about four G's. Following a brief vertical up line, the nose is pulled over into a level flight track position. Inverted level flight is maintained until the horizontal line is the same length as the vertical line, when the nose is pulled down to vertical for the third side, followed by level flight recovery. One closes the figure by flying past the original vertical line.

The horizontal lines are horizontal tracks while the vertical lines are vertical attitudes. Since the airspeed is low during the inverted flight leg, the time to fly the top line will exceed the time spent on the vertical, either going up or down. A final important factor is compensation for the wind. If the Square Loop is begun into a head wind, the top leg will take less time, as the inverted line will be flown with a tail wind. With equal length vertical legs, recovery to the entry altitude should be easy. Since missing this altitude is an easily detected error, you should be sure to get the altitude just right. The ideal Square Loop has its corners formed by Quarter Loops of the same radius, which is very difficult to do, so emphasis should be placed on at least having the same radius on the two top (slow) and bottom (fast) Quarter Loops.

THE HAMMERHEAD

No maneuver is more elegant to execute and to watch than the Hammerhead (figure VI-7). The airplane rises on a vertical line until the upward motion appears to stop, then it suddenly pivots and heads straight down, recovering at the same altitude as it began. It looks simple and it is, although it takes a good feel for the airspeed even when the airspeed is so low that the airspeed indicator has long since dropped off scale.

Many pilots are introduced to the Hammerhead early in an aerobatic curriculum, but I do not recommend this because of the risks involved if the maneuver is badly goofed. Since for-

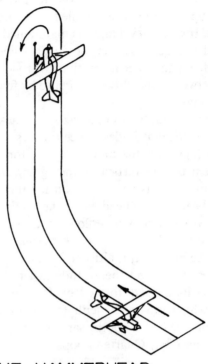

VI-7   THE HAMMERHEAD

The Hammerhead carries the airplane straight up until it almost stops, then it is pivoted by use of the rudder to begin a vertical dive.

ward control pressure at low airspeed is involved, there is the potential for accidentally entering an Inverted Spin. If the vertical up line is held too long, then an accidental Tailslide may be entered, and most airplanes are restricted from doing this maneuver.

The Hammerhead is executed by entering a full-power vertical climb (145 mph in the Decathlon). The airspeed will drop

TIMING THE PIVOT

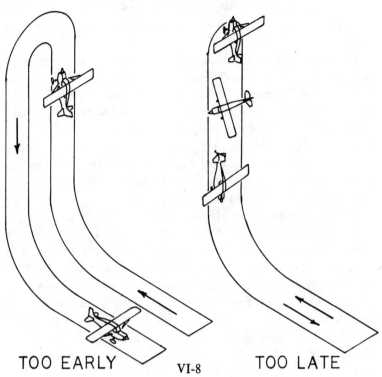

TOO EARLY   VI-8   TOO LATE

If the rudder is applied too soon the airplane flies over the top; if applied too late, the airplane will have begun to slide backwards.

rapidly and just before the airplane stops its upward motion, full left rudder is firmly applied. If timed accurately, the airplane will pivot about its vertical axis, the nose and tail swapping ends. Recovery is by a second vertical line (now diving) of the same length as the first and a Quarter Loop recovery to the entry altitude.

The timing of rudder application is critical. If you apply the rudder too soon, the airplane flies over the top in what looks like a variation of the Wingover (figure VI-8). If applied too late, the airplane starts to slide back sideways before the nose comes down to the vertical.

Power is used well into the pivot but many planes will need to have the power brought back after the pivot has started. In some planes the power will almost be at idle by the time the nose down position is reached. Power is an essential ingredient of the pivot itself, for it is the propeller slipstream blowing past the vertical tail surfaces that gives the rudder its effectiveness, as the airspeed flow is very small. If you are flying certain airplanes with small engines, you will need to initiate rudder use well before the airspeed has dropped to zero.

The challenge of the Hammerhead is to pivot at the right time and precisely about the vertical axis. That is, the airplane's wings should remain in the same plane as the nose comes around. This isn't all that easy because engine torque tends to roll the airplane to the left, precession to pitch the nose up, while the higher lift from the outside wing will tend to roll the airplane to the left. The pilot usually finds it necessary to have forward-right stick in order to keep the wings in the plane during the pivot.

THE TAILSLIDE

The Tailslide is an unlimited category maneuver that belongs in the repertoire of the quite advanced pilot who is flying a very sturdy airplane. Although not normally encountered at this point in instruction, it is covered here because this is a discussion of vertical lines. It is flown by flying the vertical up line (figure VI-9) with absolute attention to the vertical attitude and yaw (wing tip up or down) until the airplane's upward motion stops and the force of gravity begins to slide the airplane backwards. After a visible slide, usually about two fuselage lengths,

TAILSLIDES

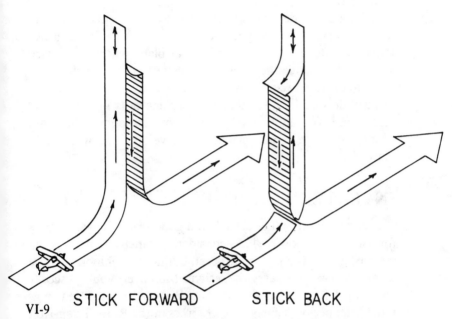

VI-9 STICK FORWARD STICK BACK

Tailslides involve flying the airplane vertically until it stops, then actually begins going backwards. The direction the control stick is moved determines which way the airplane will flop when the slide is stopped.

the elevator is moved from its neutral position, causing the airplane to *quickly* swap ends, after which the normal vertical dive recovery is made. Any deviations from neutral controls will show up in a premature reversal, a sideways tailslide or a partial roll. Since aileron and rudder are used to compensate for the disturbing torques introduced by the engine, torques should be minimized by reducing the power to idle before the airspeed drops to zero. When the slide begins, any control forces left in from the climb will be in the wrong direction as the airplane is then in a tail wind. If you do it just right, the wings will stay level as the nose reverses.

A long Tailslide can only result when the airplane is absolutely neutral. As the airplane accelerates backwards, the sensitivity to controls increases and the airplane will reverse itself very quickly. Since the Tailslide reversal can occur either nose forward or nose back, many pilots "cheat" by just a few degrees of attitude to guarantee that the airplane falls in the correct direction. If you fall through in the wrong direction, you've not simply done the maneuver badly, you've done the wrong maneuver!

INVERTED FLIGHT

Inverted flight makes clear that a good seat belt system pays for itself. Up to now we have considered maneuvers that for the most part kept the pilot in his seat, but now we'll look at those where the lap belts carry the weight. Moreover, you'll discover anything left loose in the cockpit. We've previously encountered brief periods of negative G forces in the Rolls, Loop-Roll combinations and the Square Loop, but none of these require real mastery of inverted flight techniques.

The sensations encountered in inverted flight are uncomfortable at first, but experience makes them less disconcerting. Although a pilot being introduced to inverted flight may understand what he needs to do, there is always a certain adjustment period until he does what is correct. After this adjustment, anything done inside (with positive G forces) can be done outside (with negative G forces), with practice, of course.

Unless you are flying an aircraft with absolutely symmetric airfoils and ailerons, and no incidence, your airplane will not fly as well inverted. If a high-lift airfoil is used, it will be less efficient in negative angles of attack than in positive. Nevertheless, all airplanes with inverted fuel and oil systems can be flown inverted with some degree of success. It is simply a case of orienting the airfoil to produce lift in the desired direction. In inverted level flight, one may find the airspeed to be lower than normal; the only other real difference is that when a wing comes down, it has to be pushed instead of pulled back to the horizontal.

Inverted turns take some forethought. They involve coordinated use of the controls but in opposite combinations to that in the upright turn. In the inverted turn the rudder is applied in the desired direction of turn, but the stick is moved in the opposite direction. Since aerobatic inverted turns must also have a bank angle of at least 60°, the plane will encounter at least minus two G's and the negative angle of attack will have to be increased by forward stick. At recovery to a heading, opposite rudder is used, the wing is pushed back to horizontal and the nose comes back towards the horizon. It takes some getting used to and early attempts at inverted turns will usually involve small heading changes and moderate bank angles.

OUTSIDE MANEUVERS

Pushing outside for maneuvers represents a natural dividing line for aerobatics. It is more demanding on aircraft since it requires more power for airplanes with positive incidence and high-lift airfoils. It is also more demanding on pilots in that it presents the world in a new and unnatural perspective and it is associated with a real degree of discomfort. It is possible for everyone to at least sample outside maneuvers and to decide for himself whether outside maneuvers are for him. They are clearly more demanding, and it is the pilots who have been there who most appreciate watching someone else do a series of inside and outside maneuvers equally well.

Outside maneuvers are usually approached through small

increments, for example, from high speed inverted flight pushing up to 45° lines, then to the vertical and then on over to level upright flight for a Half Outside Loop. This form of introduction to high negative G's is best, in the sense that it is easy to let up on the G loading quickly, something that cannot be done if the introduction comes in a dive. The discomfort of negative G is much like that produced by standing on your head for too long; reasons for the discomfort will be discussed later (chapter 10), when we discuss physiology. The problem is not serious; it just takes some exposure and accommodation.

Let's look at a few of the outside maneuvers that form the basis of the many possible variations. The Outside Half Loop is usually preceded by a Half Roll (155 mph in the Pitts S2A),

OUTSIDE HALF LOOP   ENGLISH BUNT

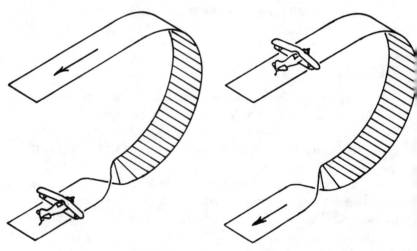

VI-10

Outside Half Loops and English Bunts are the usual introductions to large negative G loads.

quickly followed by a push of about minus three G's. All the factors we observed in the Loop will come into play here (figure VI-10), such as the decrease in G load as the airspeed decreases, which preserves the roundness of the Loop. One important difference is that the torques due to P-factor and precession will now be reversed from what we encountered in the Loop, so that it is easy to be off heading upon arrival on top.

The English Bunt is the reverse of the Immelmann, since one starts in level flight at a slow airspeed (85 mph in the Pitts S2A) and the nose is pitched forward (figure VI-10) into an Outside Half Loop with a Half Roll on the bottom as soon as the horizontal is reached. One usually remembers his first experi-

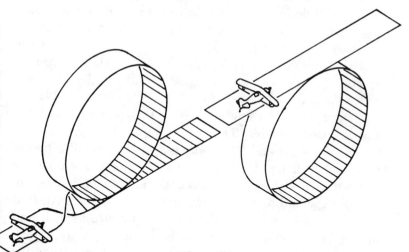

OUTSIDE LOOPS

FROM THE BOTTOM   FROM THE TOP

VI-11

Outside Loops can be started from the top or the bottom. The element of roundness is just as important as in the inside Loops.

ence with the English Bunt, for it is anything but natural to push down past the vertical with the G forces coming in and the airspeed building up. However, with repetition you'll gain the touch of pushing slow enough at the start to set a radius that can be kept and still keep the airspeed from building up too much at the bottom.

The Outside Loop can be started from the top or the bottom (figure VI-11). Starting from the bottom usually demands a preceding Half Roll and engenders a slightly greater chance of having a wing down as the push is started, but it can be done with a little less G force, since the speed can be less on the top than if you start from level flight on the top.

OUTSIDE SNAP ROLLS

The Outside Snap Roll, like the inside Snap Roll, can be done from any straight line position, upright or inverted horizontal, climbing or diving vertical. The principles are also the same, in that the Outside Snap Roll is also an autorotation maneuver, except now one is looking at large negative angles of attack. When flown from horizontal inverted flight (figure VI-12), the airplane again uses a slow airspeed (100 mph in the Pitts S2A) and low cruise power. The stick is rapidly pushed forward, stalling the wings and full rudder is applied in the direction of the desired rotation. If a faster rotation is desired, aileron in the opposite direction can be added once the rotation has begun. The precession forces we encountered in the inside Snap Roll will also be present here, in the sense that the airplane will tend to snap better to the left. This can be confusing (figure VI-12), and you may need to get a model and go back and study the lift coefficient illustration in the previous chapter. Recovery is accomplished by neutralizing the ailerons, stopping the rotation with reversed rudder and then bringing the nose down (stick back) to break the stall. It all happens fast and the observer may

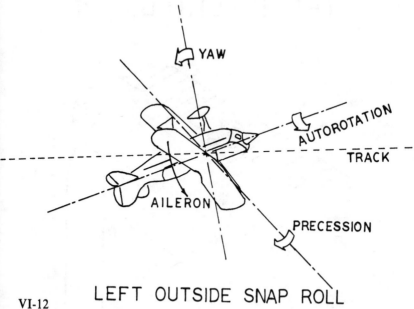

YAW

AUTOROTATION

TRACK

AILERON

PRECESSION

VI-12　　LEFT OUTSIDE SNAP ROLL

The Outside Snap Roll involves rapidly pushing about three to four negative G's. The effects of precession cause the airplane to rotate faster to the left.

not catch if the snap was inside or outside, but the pilot clearly knows, as he will encounter about negative three to four G's.

INVERTED SPINS

The Inverted Spin is as stable a flight situation as the upright Spin. Again, its basic driving force is autorotation, but this is now at large negative angles of attack. As an elementary aerobatic maneuver, it is entered as one would expect. A decelerating inverted level track ends with a full negative stall and immediate rotation by application of full rudder. It will usually

THE INVERTED SPIN

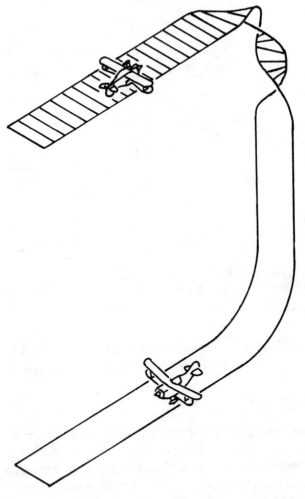

VI-13

The one-turn Inverted Spin from inverted to upright is like its upright counterpart, but it is now a reversing maneuver.

take lots of forward stick pressure to keep the wings at stall during the autorotation, especially in non-symmetric airfoil aircraft. Recovery is again by application of opposite rudder and application of back stick, to stop the rotation and unstall the wings. With recovery at the bottom to upright flight, the Inverted Spin becomes a reversing maneuver that goes from low to high airspeed (figure VI-13).

You'll find that the recovery will take less anticipation of heading than in the upright Spin, for far more rudder surface is exposed in the Inverted Spin. Figure VI-14 shows this effect. The upper structure of the tail of most airplanes is such that the

RUDDER BLOCKING IN THE SPIN

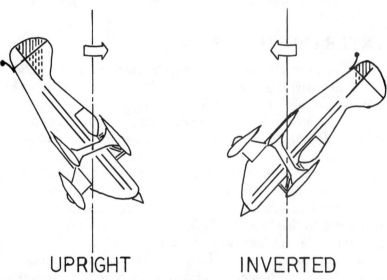

UPRIGHT   INVERTED

VI-14

The ordinary airplane recovers faster from the Inverted Spin. This is because the area blocked by the horizontal stabilizer (the shaded area) is much less in the Inverted Spin.

horizontal stabilizer shields most of the rudder in the upright Spin. It is hardly surprising that the Inverted Spin recovery is faster.

The Inverted Spin can be entered accidentally whenever forward stick pressure at low airspeed is encountered, for example, in badly executed Half Loops, Cuban Eights and Hammerheads. It is important for the beginning aerobatic pilot to have exposure to both upright and Inverted Spins prior to being turned loose for solo practice. In the confusion of a muffed maneuver, it can be difficult to tell that you are riding slightly outside instead of slightly inside. The procedures for stopping one type of spin are the ones that guarantee the other type will keep autorotating. Learn to recognize the differences and how to recover from the accidental spin in a hurry because they use up a lot of altitude quickly.

INVERTED FLAT SPINS

The Inverted Flat Spin is a simple maneuver but one to be taken seriously. It is in itself not difficult in execution or recovery, but has taken more than its share of experienced low-level pilots. Executed with a predetermined number of rotations and with ample altitude, it is a safe, stable, well-controlled aerobatic maneuver.

Consider again the principles of autorotation discussed earlier. In the ordinary Spin (either upright or inverted) the nose of the airplane is close to the vertical after the stable Spin (autorotation) has been established. The wings remain near the stall angle of attack because the flight path is nearly vertical. Up to now, we have discussed spins with the engine at idle. At idle power the effect of holding in full forward or back stick pressure does nothing more than keep the wings stalled and the Spin going.

If power is applied during a Spin, precession will immediately

INVERTED FLAT SPIN

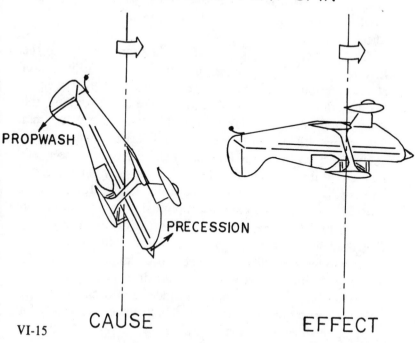

VI-15   CAUSE   EFFECT

The Inverted Flat Spin is done by adding engine power to push the tail down. The experience of riding upside down, earthward in a horizontal airplane is memorable.

become important, because a rapidly rotating propeller is now being yawed rapidly. Precession will force the nose up in a right (rudder) Inverted Spin, and it will force the nose down in a left (rudder) Inverted Spin. Not only will precession become important, the significantly increased prop wash across the elevator will tend to push the nose higher in both the upright and inverted spins. In the inverted right spin, these effects are cumulative, bringing the nose well above the vertical; in an inverted left spin the two forces approximately cancel. Understanding this, we see that it is possible to perform a Flat Spin, defined as where the airplane wings are brought to at least 45° from the vertical.

The Inverted Flat Spin is entered in the same fashion as the Inverted Spin. After the clean break of the stall and initiation of autorotation with the right rudder, power is brought back in. If this is done after about 1/2 turn of nose down rotation, the affect of Slipstream acting on the full forward elevator and Precession will be most remarkable. The nose comes up to about the horizon (in the Pitts S2A) and the rotation seems to increase. With the high rate of rotation and very flat angle, the altitude lost per turn will dramatically lessen. It will seem exactly like you are upside down on a slowly descending top and the first few Inverted Flat Spins usually leave even experienced aerobatic pilots confused about heading. Recovery is again step by step, the first is to abruptly reduce power to idle, whereupon the airplane's nose should drop into an ordinary Inverted Spin, and then opposite rudder and back stick.

Experimentation will tell how much power is needed for bringing the nose up. In many airplanes it will take full throttle. Even that will give less than full power as the engine's air scoop is now thoroughly shielded on the top side of a downward moving aircraft.

Inverted Flat Spins are to be handled with care. They should be executed in an aircraft type known to drop out of the flat position as soon as power is removed and a particular airplane whose forward Center of Gravity has been specifically determined. Moreover, it should first be done dual. Some airplanes will not bring the nose up during a left inverted spin but will begin rotating very rapidly and entering a new stable regime. Recovery may take several rotations to stop the spin even after power is removed and opposite rudder is applied. Those few extra rotations can seem to take several months if you expect the usual immediate response!

In this chapter we have covered many new maneuvers, maneuvers that might be considered advanced since they involve different conditions (even in their simplest forms) from those encountered in the most basic positive maneuvers. They are a mixed bag as far as difficulty is concerned, for some of them are learned early, while others are usually attacked by the journeyman aerobatic pilot. They share many elements, however, and this order of presentation can be defended as logical for understanding them, even if it is not suitable for a training course syllabus.

7
Maneuvers-
Compound

IN THIS CHAPTER we will describe those maneuvers that combine elements of different maneuvers and represent significant variations on maneuvers discussed previously. But first, a minor digression.

At some point in your aerobatic flying, perhaps when a single-seat aircraft is all that is available, you will find yourself in the position of being your own teacher. In this case, extreme caution should be observed and the maneuvers should be well thought out beforehand. This type of learning can be done if it builds on a solid base of experience and knowledge developed in early flight training, but the introduction to a new flight regime should be done dual, in a proven aircraft. There are enough training centers in the United States within reach of any serious pilot who wants to get into a new area of aerobatics. A few hours with a professional can save many hours of trial and error on one's own. All of this can be said in another way: any new area of aerobatics should be introduced by dual instruction, whether it is the first Loop or the first Inverted Flat Spin.

AVALANCHE

This British term describes a Loop with a Snap Roll on top. It is done in the same way as an ordinary Loop, with all of the usual attention to roundness, but with about 5 mph higher entry speed. As the airplane approaches the top of the Loop (figure VII-1), an inside Snap Roll is begun, with the timing

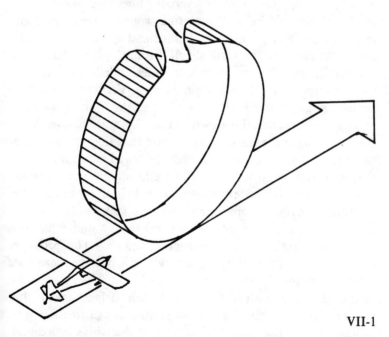

AVALANCHE

VII-1

The Avalanche, or Snap Roll on top of the Loop, is an added challenge. It should be exactly centered and blend in smoothly with the Loop.

such that the Snap Roll is exactly centered on the top. If timed correctly, the nose will come down smoothly in the recovery from the Snap Roll into the continuation of the Loop. From then on, it is flown as in a Round Loop, since the extra speed carried into the top of the Loop has been absorbed in the Snap Roll. The clock angle at which the Snap Roll is begun depends on the aircraft type; in the Pitts Special it is about 15° ahead.

VERTICAL ROLLS

Vertical rolls are a distinguishing feature in advanced flying and form a major portion of all international competition maneuvers. In our discussion of vertical lines, we saw that the length of the climbing vertical line would depend on many factors, especially the entry technique and speed and the power/weight ratio. In the vertical roll the airplane will have even less vertical penetration because the aileron deflections used to roll the airplane produce additional drag. Vertical rolls can be as little as a Quarter Roll or as much as the limit of the most muscular international competition machine, about five. All of these rolls have the feature in common that they must be centered on the vertical line and must be true longitudinal rolls, that is, variations from the vertical attitude are not allowed.

This on-axis, vertical rotation is more difficult in the climbing vertical roll because reference objects are lacking. In this case one must look to the side to pick up the ground references needed to stop the roll on a particular heading. This produces a natural tendency to drop a wing, which is much easier to see from the ground than it is from the pilot's seat. The yaw component of the prop wash that acts on the tail surfaces means that you may need to make a certain continuous correction with rudder to keep the nose straight up and the wings horizontal. This correction will change as the airspeed drops. The adverse yaw that characterizes the entry to an ordinary level turn will

VERTICAL ROLL

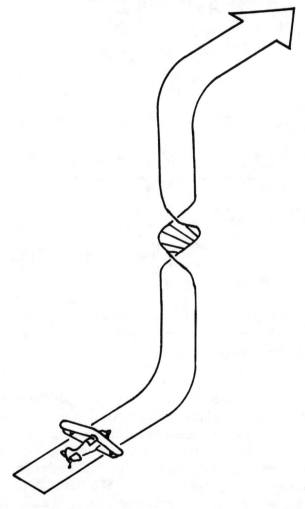

VII-2

The climbing Vertical Roll requires lots of entry speed and horsepower. It is the truest form of roll: since the wings are not producing lift, it is done exactly on-axis.

YAW FORCES
RIGHT VERTICAL ROLL

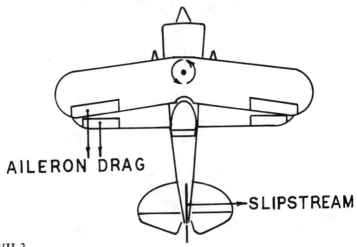

AILERON DRAG

SLIPSTREAM

VII-3

There are two major forces tending to make the airplane drop a wing during the right vertical roll. The balance of these depends on speed, power, design and engine speed.

also cause the need for corrective rudder. Adverse yaw is caused by the additional drag of the downward aileron as compared with the upward aileron. In the case of a vertical roll to the left, some left rudder will be needed to keep the wings horizontal and the nose pinned to the vertical, while right rudder compensates for a right roll. Since Slipstream torque will always be pushing the left wing tip down, less rudder should be needed in the left vertical roll. And since the rolls must be centered in position, the straight line above the roll will take much longer to fly than the lower straight line, which is done at a far higher airspeed.

HUMPTY BUMPS

This peculiar name covers a family of maneuvers characterized by a vertical line with climbing half rolls, a Half Loop over to a diving vertical line followed by recovery to horizontal flight at the same altitude as the entry. In this case, all the usual quality criteria for the individual components apply, including level entry and exit, constant radius transitions at the bottom, half roll centered on the vertical line and maintenance of heading throughout. Since the airspeed is very low after the half roll, the Half Loop on top can be smaller than that for the Quarter Loops on the bottom, but its radius must be constant and the airplane must fly over the top, not just swap ends.

The Humpty Bump family has many members; they can be

HUMPTY BUMPS

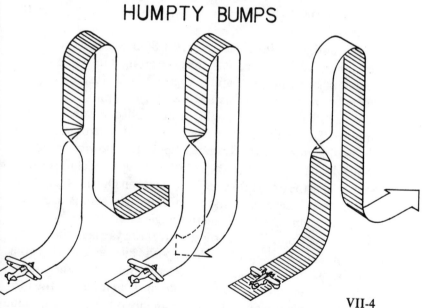

VII-4

There are many varieties of Humpty Bumps, three of which are shown here. They share the same basic elements but in different combinations.

entered and/or exited from upright and inverted flight, and the Half Loop on top can be either inside or outside (figure VII-4). Such variation offers many possible combinations for the aircraft with good vertical climb performance. The possibilities become even greater when one considers that the half rolls can be half of a Slow Roll, a Snap Roll or a Hesitation Roll and the pilot can substitute one-quarter or three-quarter turn rolls for the half roll.

CROSSOVER SPINS

Thus far we have considered only upright Spins entered from upright flight and Inverted Spins entered from inverted flight, but if we stopped at these straightforward approaches, things would be dull indeed. It is possible to enter the Inverted Spin from upright flight and vice versa, which are called here the Crossover Spins.

The upright to inverted Crossover Spin begins in power-off, level-decelerating flight, with the nose brought up to higher and higher positive angles of attack (figure VII-5). Just as the point of stall is reached, full forward elevator is applied and held in firmly, full rudder is brought in and full opposite aileron is applied. This most peculiar combination of control forces produces the entry to the Inverted Spin. The slow airspeed obtained by deceleration to the point of the upright stall is necessary to give the drop into a spin instead of an Outside Snap Roll. Full forward elevator at the point of upright stall is necessary for establishing the high negative angle of attack necessary for an Inverted Spin. The full rudder gives the yawing motion that leads to autorotation, while the opposite aileron smoothly rolls the aircraft into position for the Inverted Spin. Once the autorotation is established, the aileron into the spin increases the turn rate. Recovery is similar to that from any other Inverted Spin, that is, a smooth stop on heading, vertical line and recovery to level flight.

CROSSOVER SPIN

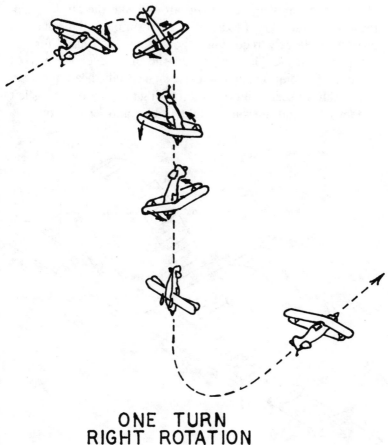

ONE TURN
RIGHT ROTATION

VII-5

The Crossover Spin shown is one inverted rotation with an upright entry and exit. It takes a sharp eye to tell it from the ordinary Spin. The pilot knows the big difference in the way it is flown.

The reciprocal procedure applies for the inverted to upright Crossover Spin, except the same sense of rudder and aileron is used. You can study either of these maneuvers beforehand, but use a model: moving your hand around like the airplane can twist something. Try it. Basically, it is a simple and mechanical procedure, largely requiring a good sense of timing for the entry. If you are planning to do this maneuver for a fixed fraction of a rotation and come out on a specific heading, it can be a real head-scratching situation trying to figure out if it is left rudder and right aileron or right rudder and left aileron!

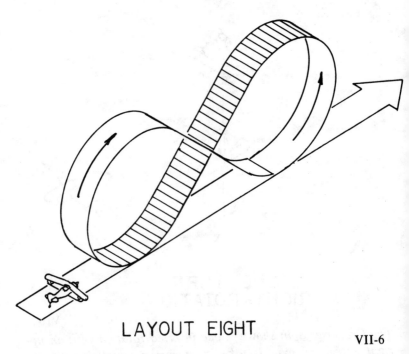

LAYOUT EIGHT

VII-6

The Layout Eight is really an inside-outside horizontal eight. When flown exactly right, the loops are of equal size and the lines cross in the middle.

HORIZONTAL EIGHTS

The basic Cuban Eight (which is two combined Half Cubans) has a set of related advanced maneuvers. Although complete eights, they do not involve repetitions. The Layout Eight is a Half Cuban without the half roll, followed by three-fourths of an Outside Loop and an upright recovery (figure VII-6). The Outside Eight is related, but involves a half roll on the first 45° line (figure VII-7) to prevent repetition and to bring the airplane into position for an upright recovery. There are many other horizontal eights involving upright and inverted entries

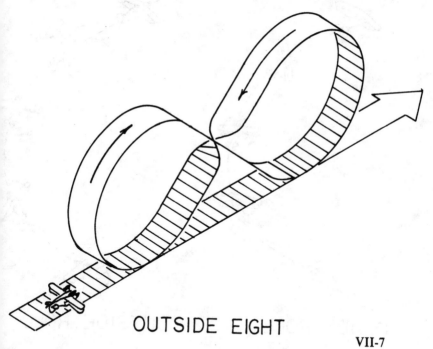

OUTSIDE EIGHT

VII-7

The Outside Eight has inverted flight until the last part. The Half Roll should be placed at the spot where the second straight line will be intersecting.

and exits, inside and outside partial loops and fraction Rolls, Snap Rolls and Hesitation Rolls. They all share a difference of execution on the two sides, head wind-tail wind corrections to the lines and loops and careful attention to placement of the half rolls.

ONE ROLL 90° TURN

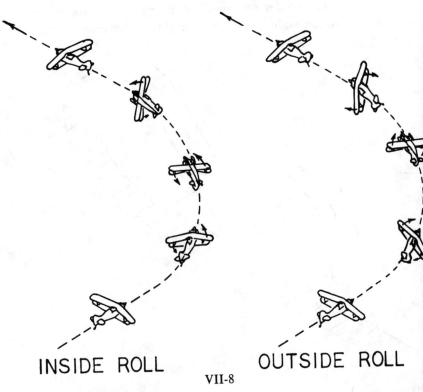

INSIDE ROLL   OUTSIDE ROLL

VII-8

Rolling Turns can be done with the rolls to the inside or outside. The outside roll is considered more difficult, although many of its elements are the same.

ROLLING TURNS

Rolling Turns are not difficult, but they can be very, very busy. They combine two basic maneuvers of the Turn with the Roll and, of course, many combinations are possible in terms of number of rolls, inverted or upright entry, 90°, 180°, or 360° heading changes and rolls to the inside or outside.

Let's walk through the first 90° of an Upright, Four Roll 360° Turn with the roll to the inside. The entry speed is that for the roll. There will be two key positions, the 45° heading point, at which we'll be inverted, and the 90° point where we'll be back to upright. We'll assume that the maneuver is being done with rolls and turns to the left. As the left turn is begun the roll is

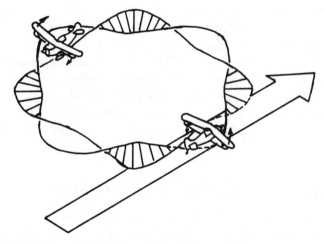

FOUR ROLL 360° TURN
VII-9

The Four Roll 360° Turn is about the busiest maneuver for the aerobatic pilot. There are eight fundamental headings to be met with the wings level. Needless to say, the control forces and direction are continuously changing.

continued and held in at full aileron throughout. At the first knife-edge position we'll need lots of top right rudder to maintain constant altitude and back elevator to keep the turn going. At the 45° heading position we'll be in slightly nose-high inverted flight (stick slightly forward) with the turn being continued by strong right rudder. At the second knife-edge position we'll have lots of top (left) rudder and the turn rate will be determined by forward elevator control. At the 90° point we're back to upright flight with wings level and rolling right into the next segment of the four-turn maneuver. The same sequence can be followed with the turns to the outside, that is, left roll with right turn and vice versa.

The maneuver demands application of all the fundamentals of the roll and both upright and inverted turns. It is not particularly uncomfortable although the normal G range will be plus two G's to minus two G's, encountered in short order. Of course, orientation can be a problem. The United States national champion got ahead of himself at the world competition in 1978 and finished his four turns after only 270°, knocking himself out of a solid first place and into the also-rans for that flight. Multiple rolling turns can go wrong at so many places that it is unusual for competitors to voluntarily include them at judged flying.

TORQUE ROLLS AND LOMCEVAKS

The Torque Rolls and Lomcevaks are breathtaking to watch and are rather recently developed aerobatic maneuvers. Probably nothing else characterizes the enormous flexibility of the modern propeller-driven aerobatic airplane than these two maneuvers.

The Torque Roll first made its appearance at the World Aerobatics Championship held in France in 1972, when Charlie Hillard of the USA team astounded the participants and judges.

During his four-minute freestyle flight he did the impossible, it was thought. Now the Torque Roll is used by many unlimited category pilots. This present popularity emphasizes Hillard's achievement, for it shows that the machines could do it, the maneuver simply awaited a skilled, innovative pilot.

The Torque Roll is executed by first performing a left vertical roll, usually entered with lots of extra airspeed to allow multiple rolls up for dramatic effect. Unlike the previous vertical rolls, in this case we leave in full aileron deflection as the airspeed drops to zero. Eventually the airplane stops rising (but is still rolling) and then begins to reverse, just like the tailslide, except now the plane is rolling! This falling direction roll is continued until the airplane falls off the vertical line or power is reduced and an ordinary tailslide reversal and recovery is performed. The right hand torque of the spinning propeller, which has been left at full power, is what continues the airplane's roll to the left at low and even zero airspeeds. A high powered, short wingspan plane like the single place Pitts does not require reversing the aileron deflection direction upon the airplane starting to drop, although this will increase the rate of roll on the way down. Reversing aileron direction is a necessity on most other planes, as the backward airflow will otherwise counteract the propeller torque.

The key to success in the Torque Roll is recognizing and maintaining the vertical line, otherwise the nose will wallow around on the way up, the vertical penetration will be reduced, and, most seriously, the plane won't pivot on its tail upon starting to fall. One must also be sure that the tail assembly is very strong, since high reverse speeds can be reached. The pilot must be experienced enough to quickly recognize and recover from the many possible accidental exits from this maneuver, which include the inverted flat spin.

Lomcevak is a Czech word for stiff drink or drunken stagger, the latter being an adequate description of the maneuver. It is

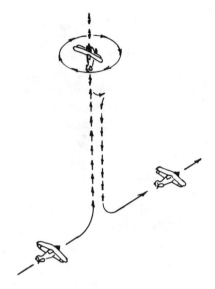

TORQUE ROLL

VII-10

The torque roll begins with a maximum rate vertical roll which continues even when the aircraft stops and reverses itself! The rolling portion is usually followed by a tailslide.

actually a family of maneuvers developed in Czechoslovakia in the 1950s by former World Champion Ladislav Bezák and his colleagues. Although these maneuvers have long technical descriptions, the important common feature is the tumble, where the airplane appears to rapidly rotate about the pitch axis. This tumble is produced by the propeller gyroscopic precession discussed in Chapter VI when we talked about Outside Snap Rolls. In the Pitts, the maneuver is started with an Outside Snap Roll at full power, using right rudder, left aileron, and forward stick. In this combination the yawing forces cause the nose to keep pitching forward. If the maneuver is begun on a nearly vertical or inverted climbing 45° line, the airplane will rapidly lose airspeed and the forward motion will drop to nearly zero. When this near zero speed situation is reached, the airplane's motion is dominated by torque induced roll, yaw from propwash flowing over the rudder, and gyroscopic precession. The airplane will then tumble at the top of the maneuver. This tumbling motion will continue until aerodynamic forces again dominate and the airplane drops down to a new state. If the control forces are left in and the power is still full, this is likely to be an inverted flat spin. All this in a matter of seconds! It cannot be overemphasized that this maneuver should only be attempted by pilots who are thoroughly familiar with climbing Outside Snap Rolls, who are not subject to disorientation, and who can immediately recognize and recover from the inverted flat spin.

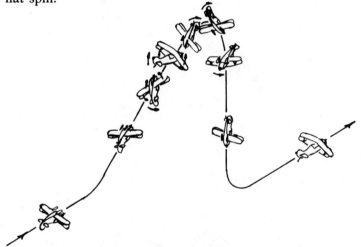

VII-11 LOMCEVAK

The particular Lomcevak shown here starts from inverted climbing flight but has the feature common to all Lomcevaks, an apparent end-over-end tumble.

Since this maneuver relies on propeller gyroscopic precession to move the entire airplane, the stresses on the propeller are higher than any other maneuver we've discussed. The incidence of propeller failures and even separation from the engine has been so high that most pilots don't attempt the maneuver, this group including many pilots whose skill level would make it an ordinary and safe maneuver.

8
Aresti–The Hieroglyphics of Aerobatics

ABOUT FIVE THOUSAND years ago the residents along the Nile River had a developing and sophisticated society, but its growth was limited. It could only pass along information by word of mouth. There arose a system of making marks that conveyed an unambiguous meaning to any reader. This ability evolved in response to the need to do business, to send such messages as, "Ship seven fatted calves and three rams, and bill to my account" by even the most forgetful slave. That is, the Egyptians developed the ability to read and write. The earliest form of writing was strictly pictorial. If you meant three fatted calves, that's what you drew. Obviously, this representation could go only so far, for it couldn't represent such concepts as, "Bill to my account." The next step was to stylize the pictures so that anyone, not just artists, could write. The last step was to take the sounds from the early words and put them together simply as sounds, which could build new words. All of a sudden, any word that could be pronounced could be printed, even if only

121

with an apparently meaningless combination of pictures. This pictographic form of writing was called hieroglyphics. We are in the early, pictorial writing phase of aerobatics and the first dictionary has been written by the Spaniard, José L. Aresti. It has quickly become the *lingua franca* of the aerobatic world and for good reason.

When the first aerobatic pilots described their maneuvers, they undoubtedly did it with models or the most convenient item, the extended flat hand. This technique works fine if you are face to face with your audience or if you are a sufficiently skillful and patient artist to draw each phase of your maneuver. But the hand or drawn presentation quickly becomes awkward when describing a sequence of maneuvers. An improvement on this representation is the ribbon method, which we have used so far in this book. However, it doesn't work all that well for a sequence and it simply cannot make its meaning utterly clear. For example, the Roll and the Snap Roll either require additional comments or an extremely skilled artist. If we jump back to the analogy with the ancient Egyptians, at the beginning it was hard to distinguish between a fatted calf and a calf for fattening. The use of the ribbon method of representation essentially disappeared when Senor Aresti published his "Aerocriptographic System." Even this language isn't perfect, because it has not grown to include new maneuvers (concepts) for which new symbols (words) have been generated. However, it does represent a concise, unambiguous way of representing almost all aerobatic maneuvers and it should be understood by all aerobatics enthusiasts.

Aresti divided aerobatic maneuvers into nine families, in which each member of a family shares certain basic characteristics. He grouped them in this order:

1. Lines and Lines plus Angles
2. Horizontal Turns

3. Vertical Turns
4. Spins
5. Hammerheads
6. Tailslides
7. Loops
8. Rolls
9. Half Rolls plus Half Loops

Since the underlying motive of the Aresti Aerocriptographic System is to have absolute clarity in describing a maneuver, each of these families has numerous members, with some much larger than others. Likewise, there needs to be a specific name for each maneuver and maneuvers that look similar should have similar names. He accomplished these goals by breaking down the families into sub-families of finer and finer steps and each time a finer subdivision is made, another number is added to the designation. Consider the "pedigree" of one particular maneuver, the Outside Loop entered from level inverted flight and finishing in level inverted flight. All loops are Family 7, all Round Loops are 7.1, all full circle round loops are 7.1.1 and finally, the subdivision of 7.1.1.1 is given to our maneuver. Confusing? Perhaps, but consider the alternatives, especially at an international contest.

For each maneuver, Aresti developed a shorthand method of representing the way in which it should be flown. The basic elements of this shorthand are shown in figure VIII-1. These elements taken together can define thousands of maneuvers, but it is essential that a few subtleties be observed. Consider the next set of drawings. The start of each maneuver has a small filled circle and the end has a line. For the vertical slow rolls, the direction of flight on which the roll is located is determined as if the curve was being drawn to represent a swept-wing plane. On the Snap Rolls the barb indicates the direction of flight when the Snap is done. Points need to be shown on the Hesita-

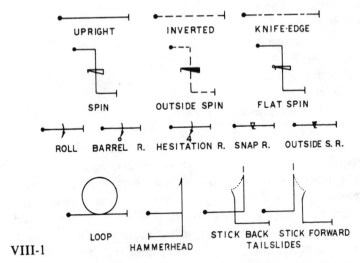

VIII-1

The most common elements of Aresti. The line symbols are shown, together with the common name for the maneuver.

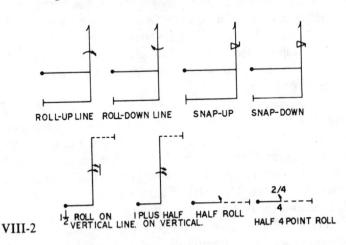

VIII-2

There are many subtle points in writing the correct symbol for a maneuver. These small differences indicate different maneuvers.

tion Rolls, as they otherwise resemble Slow Rolls. Finally, maneuvers that are continuous need to be connected by a thin line, to distinguish them from similar but separate maneuvers.

A sample from each Aresti family is shown (figure VIII-3), except for Families 1 and 3, which are not used in competition aerobatics. The figure mainly touches on a few of the many possible maneuvers, but has been selected to show the basic features that will be encountered in drawing most maneuvers. For illustration, we also show the ribbon representation together with its Aresti symbol for a few maneuvers. It should be obvious that the Aresti method is much easier to draw and is clearer. When a sequence is put together, it may be necessary to take artistic liberties, to artificially spread the figures so that they don't overlap, but this can be done using common sense as a guide. The most common set of maneuvers that are drawn one way and flown another are the Reverse Half Cubans, which are drawn with a vertical line on the back side but flown as a constant radius five-eighths loop (figure VIII-4).

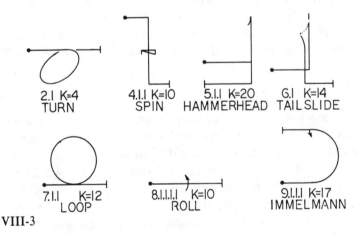

VIII-3

A few common Aresti symbols are shown, together with their catalog numbers, common name and difficulty value (K Factor).

VIII-4

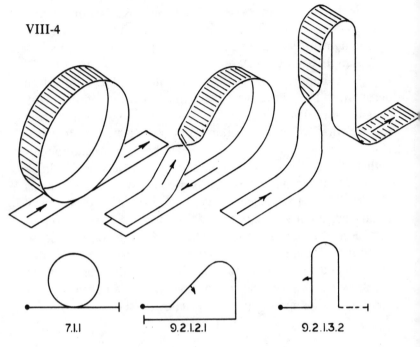

Most of the Aresti symbols closely follow the shape of the maneuver, but maneuver 9.2.1.2.1 is a good example of one that does not.

When Senor Aresti defined each maneuver, he also assigned a difficulty factor. This difficulty factor is called the K factor. For example, the simple Loop is designated 7.1.1 and has a K factor of 12 (12 K), while the Eight Sided Loop is 7.4.2 and is 22 K. Usually the K factor closely approximates the difficulty in performing a maneuver, but every pilot will find some exceptions due to his own predilection for a given maneuver or hangups about others. In the case of compound maneuvers, the overall K value is the sum of the K values of the parts. These

K values will become important when we consider the scoring of maneuvers.

As we mentioned before, the Aresti designation does have certain limitations. The primary fault is its inflexibility. Since Aresti's work, some new maneuvers have been added to the repertoire of unlimited pilots, but these do not appear in the catalog. These may be understandable for such maneuvers as the Lomcevak, which are difficult to describe concisely. This limitation is less acceptable for the Torque Rolls, in which a multiple vertical slow roll is continued well into the reversal of direction on top before swapping ends. The problem is solvable, but would require Aresti to come out with a revised edition of his catalog or to delegate authority to an international committee. Some of the maneuvers that are in this catalog are not realistic, such as 9.2.3.3.1 (a Humpty Bump with half of a vertical Barrel Roll) or 8.1.2.1.9 (a triple Super Slow Roll). The former can't be done as it would put the airplane 40° off axis while going up. The latter could only be done in an airplane flying slower than 55 mph, as each single Super Slow Roll must take at least 15 seconds. A final limitation is the fact that a few maneuvers may be flown in one way but are two different maneuvers in the Aresti Catalog and have different K values. An example is the Quarter Roll on a Vertical Line (8.1.1.1.4, 19 K) and the Quarter Four Point Hesitation Roll on a Vertical Line (8.2.2.11.4, 20 K), which are flown in exactly the same way. Rules for composing a free style sequence only allow use of the lower K versions.

Finally, it is not always clear how the maneuvers were intended to be flown, as in the example of Reverse Half Cuban (9.2.1.2.1) discussed above. Despite these few problems, Aresti is the best language we have in aerobatics; an ancient Egyptian scribe would have been proud of Senor Aresti.

9

Building Sequences— Tying It All Together

THE MANEUVERS we have discussed so far have been individual maneuvers and we concentrated our attention on how they were flown with no consideration about what preceded or followed. Likewise, our emphasis has been on basic performance and not on the many possible errors and pitfalls that prevent perfection in aerobatics. In this chapter we'll emphasize how to tie single maneuvers together and how to bring performance up to the best possible level.

SEQUENCES

Our armchair flying has enjoyed, up until now, two great freedoms, liberty to control the entry speeds exactly on the optimum values and the ability to start and stop the maneuvers without regard to position with respect to the ground. These freedoms are lost to a real degree when one wants to do a close knit set of maneuvers (a sequence) and to keep this sequence

128

over a certain piece of real estate. If forethought is given to composing a sequence and if it is flown with care, we won't compromise our previous freedoms much, but if forethought and care are abandoned, the maneuvers won't turn out right and an astonishing amount of territory will be covered.

The key to tying maneuvers together is understanding entry and exit speeds. We have talked mostly about entry speeds, but it should be obvious that the exit speeds can be very different. In such maneuvers as the Loop and Hammerhead, the exit speeds will be almost the same as the entry speeds if the altitudes are exactly the same. Equal altitudes usually mean nearly equal speeds, but this is not always entirely so. If an airplane has sufficient engine power to reach the entry speed without diving, and power is used throughout the maneuver, then a return to original altitude will also mean a return to the same airspeed. However, if it is necessary to dive for entry speed, then

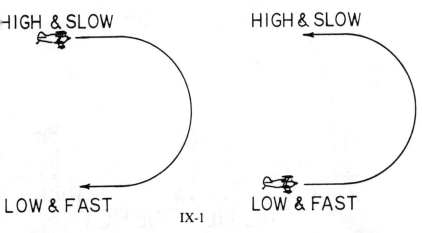

IX-1

In some maneuvers the altitude and airspeed will unavoidably change. The skilled pilot tries to obtain the right combination. For example, if you try starting the left-hand maneuver high and fast, you'll end up low and too fast.

the exit speed at the same altitude will usually be slower, even if power was used throughout. This means that lower power airplanes require working at the slowest possible entry speeds in order to minimize the amount of diving done between maneuvers.

Some maneuvers, like the Spin, start at low airspeed and high altitude but end with high airspeed and low altitude; others, like the Immelmann start with high airspeed and low altitude but end with low airspeed and high altitude. These relationships

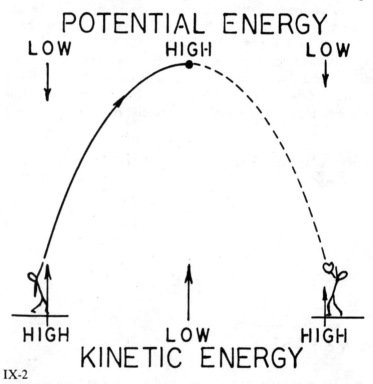

IX-2

Objects moved against the force of gravity trade their kinetic energy for potential energy. This trade applies whether one is talking about a baseball or an airplane.

result from the fact that in these maneuvers one is trading kinetic energy (the energy of a moving object) for potential energy (the energy that an object has as a result of its altitude). All moving objects possess kinetic energy, which increases quickly with airspeed. Kinetic energy is the reason it is difficult to brake a fast-moving car. All objects, moving and non-moving, possess potential energy, the amount depending on how much work it took to get the object where it is. If we throw a ball up into the air (figure IX-2), it leaves our hand with high kinetic energy and low potential energy. When it reaches its highest point, the upward kinetic energy has been depleted by working against gravity and has now been stored as potential energy. As the ball drops back to our hand, the potential energy is converted back to kinetic energy. It is caught at almost the original speed, but not quite, for some energy has been lost due to air drag. In a maneuvering airplane, the same considerations apply. If there is enough energy supplied by the engine to overcome aerodynamic drag, then we can trade altitude and airspeed back and forth until the fuel is used up.

In the best combinations of maneuvers, the exit speed of one maneuver closely matches the optimum entry airspeed of the next maneuver, with only a short period of acceleration or deceleration necessary in between. Consider this alphabetical list of maneuvers: Immelmann, Loop, Snap Roll, Spin, Split S. Flying them in fast pace in this order would be nearly impossible in most airplanes, for the slow exit speed of the Immelmann would not be matched to the start of the Loop, and the high exit speed of the Loop would be too great for the Snap Roll, and so on (figure IX-3). Probably the optimum combination is Spin, Immelmann, Snap Roll, Split S and Loop (figure IX-4). You will unavoidably lose altitude in this set, since there are two descending maneuvers (Spin and Split S) and only one climbing maneuver (the Immelmann).

AN AWKWARD SEQUENCE

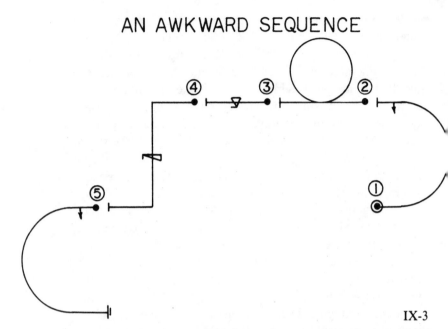

IX-3

Maneuvers must be combined in a flow in which the exit speed for one matches the entry speed for the next. This sequence is arranged alphabetically; it would be very difficult to fly in close combination.

Building a sequence requires experience in your airplane, patience and imagination. The more maneuvers in your bag of tricks, the easier it will be to tie things together. Composing a completely free sequence is easy, but when certain "rules" are imposed, composition becomes more challenging. We'll see later that this challenge prevails in all levels of American aerobatic flying, for certain types of maneuvers must be included in each level; in fact, the included maneuvers help to define the levels of competition.

THE CORRECT SEQUENCE

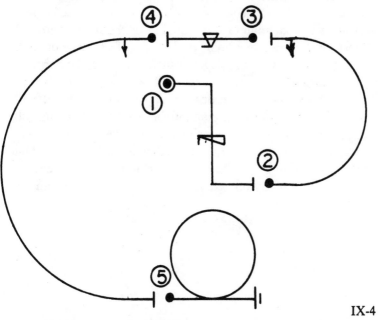

IX-4

The set of maneuvers shown in the previous figure are reordered here to allow a smooth flow from one maneuver to the next.

CROSSWIND CORRECTIONS

Another liberty that we have allowed ourselves in our arm-chair flying has been to fly only in calm conditions or winds directly into the maneuvers. Obviously, such liberties will usually not be the case in actual flight and the effects of a crosswind quickly show up when one starts flying sequences. That negligible 10-mph crosswind component can carry you 4400 feet after five minutes of flying, well away from where you wanted to be and nearly out of sight of observers. The aerobatic pilot will need to know how to correct for crosswind components as well as head and tail wind components and to make these corrections in ways that maintain the quality of the maneuvers.

Most maneuvers are planar, that is, if perfectly executed all parts fall on the same flat surface, a surface that can be horizontal (such as a rolling turn) or vertical (a Loop, for example). Crosswind components can destroy the apparent symmetry of a maneuver in the vertical plane if the wind is strong and no corrections are applied. The principles involved in the corrections are the same as those used in calculating headings when flying cross country. The heading one assumes is into the wind by an amount directly related to the crosswind strength and the airplane's airspeed.

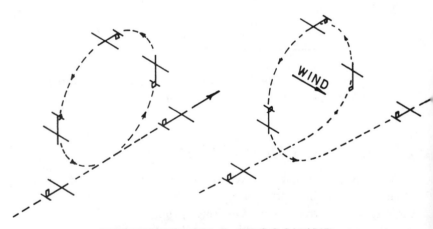

EFFECTS OF A CROSSWIND

IX-5

A crosswind can turn a perfectly flown Loop into a spiral if the same heading is used throughout.

This simple theory becomes a little more complex when applied to aerobatic flying because the direction and the airspeed change rapidly. Consider a Loop being flown with a crosswind from the left. An observer viewing this loop from a downwind position (figure IX–5) would see the airplane exit the loop higher than the entry altitude if no crosswind correction was applied. As the maneuver is begun, the heading will need to be only slightly left since the airspeed is high, but when the air-

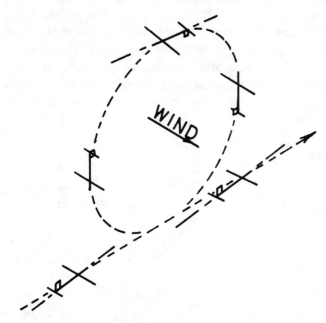

CROSSWIND CORRECTIONS

IX-6

Crosswind corrections are necessary for flying the exact figures. The angle into the wind depends on the airspeed. In the Loop shown here, the correction on the top is much larger than that on the bottom, where the airspeed is high.

plane is inverted on top, the correction must be further left at a larger angle since the airspeed will be quite low. Such corrections seem incompatible with the demand that perfect maneuvers be flown with respect to ground headings; however, if the deviations are obviously for crosswind correction and they are appropriate in direction and amount, then such corrections reveal an even higher mastery of aerobatic flying.

Even if you continuously and smoothly apply crosswind corrections, it is often impossible to fly a complex sequence over a limited area of ground. It is then advisable to include Crosswind maneuvers in your sequence. Such inclusion allows the individual maneuvers to be flown more nearly as they are drawn, which is easier, and then to make the position corrections as parts of specific maneuvers. These crosswind correction maneuvers and combinations work in one of two ways: dis-

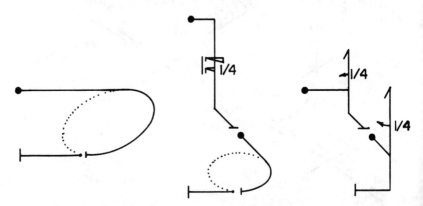

CROSSWIND CORRECTION MANEUVERS

IX-7

Crosswind maneuvers and combinations can be used to correct position changes due to crosswind without having to fly corrections within each individual maneuver.

placement of position to the left or right while changing heading by 180° or by two changes of heading of 90° (figure IX-7). An example of the first type is the 180° turn, which simply relocates the aircraft to one side after completion. A simple example of the second type is a one and one-quarter turn Spin followed by a 90° turn, a combination that can produce a considerable position correction, depending on the gap between the two maneuvers.

In a lengthy sequence more than one crosswind correction combination is included so that the continuous crosswind corrections can be kept small. This is simple when there is a wind, but in the event that it is calm, they'll have to be flown in opposite and compensating directions.

When you include crosswind correction within individual maneuvers and within a sequence, you add a thinking requirement to the requirement to fly. Often the two do not come together, which is hardly surprising since changes occur quickly, and it is sometimes hard to distinguish between position changes due to bad flying and those due to wind. The distinction *can* be made: it simply takes experience in lots of different flying conditions.

PERFECTING ONE'S PERFORMANCE

The saying "practice makes perfect" carries a lot of wisdom, but practicing the wrong things does not lead to perfection. A solo pilot can develop his flying techniques until things feel "just right"; however, many situations feel one way, but look another. Climbing vertical lines are an excellent example, in which the beginning pilot just can't believe that the nose has to be that far back, with all that weight on his shoulder and back. To gain that special competitive edge, it is best to get a keen-eyed observer on the ground, possibly another pilot, but certainly someone who knows what things to watch for. Let's call that observer The Coach. If you are aiming for competition

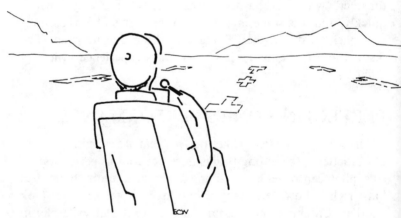

IX-8

*The Coach is an essential ingredient of successful aerobatic com-
petition training. The Coach is shown here armed with a flight
sequence sheet, tape recorder and good eyes. (Drawing by Eliza
Walbridge)*

flying or other observed conditions, what counts is how the flying looks from the ground, not how it looks from inside the airplane. That inertial gyroscope you borrowed and are carrying along just this once may tell you that you are really flying a 40° line, but if it looks like a 45° line, then it *is* correct. This is what makes it essential to have a good Coach.

The Coach is really only useful if your flying is consistent. If you do a given maneuver in several ways in several attempts, then the opinion of The Coach isn't worth much, unless you have a phenomenal memory and can reconstruct each maneuver individually. By first training to the point of consistency, you should be able to easily relate observed results to pilot technique. There is always the danger of practicing something the wrong way until your bad habits can become hard to break, so it is wise to get help as soon as you are on top of each maneuver.

When one is working on individual maneuvers, it is possible to make good use of two-way radio contact, to quickly correct mistakes and peak up one's performance; however, when one is flying sequences, some form of record, which can be reviewed upon landing, should be made on the ground. The best device for this is the portable tape recorder. The Coach should know what maneuvers are to be flown and should keep up a constant description of what he sees, so the pilot can tell just where the comments apply. Five minutes of recorded engine roar punctuated by the isolated comments "Settled," "Tucked 10°" and "Off heading 5°" will be of little aid to anyone. The Coach should tell what he sees the pilot doing so that the comments can be accurately located in the sequence. When you employ such techniques, your progress can be rapid and you'll be surprised with the results. Of course, the ideal thing is to have a line of qualified Coaches all down there, averaging out one another's mistakes, but the biggest step is getting that first Coach.

REFERENCE AIDES

Aerobatics are flown using all the information our senses can gather, but most of the information is visual and our vision is largely restricted to the view from the cockpit. This means that we judge our attitude with respect to parts of the airframe. This is best done if your eyes are close to the primary axes of the airplane and there are good references on the plane. For example, if you are flying the Pitts, it is usually argued that you should sit as low as possible (nearer the longitudinal axis), looking out over that long flat cowling. Many pilots can't get into this position without resorting to imitation of a pretzel, which is the second natural advantage of the smaller pilot (the first is that they usually weigh less and get better climb performance).

Airplanes aren't normally built with natural reference lines that allow you to set up exact 45° and 90° lines in climbs and dives, nor do they have airspeed indicators that register when you are going very slow or even backwards. Many pilots correct for these limitations by drawing reference lines on their interwing I struts or even by making frames that project directly out from their line of sight when looking sideways. A final aid, less frequently seen, is the low-cost, low-speed airspeed indicator. This is usually a piece of yarn, in contrasting color, taped by the forward end to the I strut, where it is out of the prop wash. At high airspeeds, it will be stretched out in length and oscillating rapidly. At low airspeeds, far below where the Pitot-driven cockpit instrument drops off scale, its stiffness and rate of motion tell you how much airspeed is left. This can be useful in timing Hammerheads and Tailslides. Since this airspeed indicator reads both positive and negative speeds, you'll see it pointed upwards in the Tailslide before you feel the rapid downward acceleration by gravity.

All of these aids are just supplements to using all of the

visual, kinesthetic and aural information available to you. They are useful for training, but in the end what counts is how the maneuvers look from the ground. The only way to measure your performance in the cockpit is through the feedback from a coach on the ground.

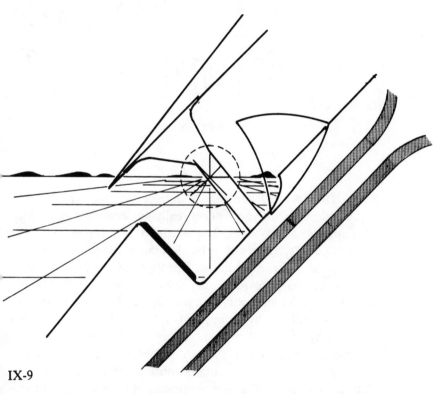

IX-9

This cockpit view of a biplane in a 45° climb attitude (with the pilot removed) shows reference aids within the dashed circle. When the reference lines are parallel to the horizon, the attitude should be just right. The wavy string is the low-speed airspeed indicator described in the text.

10
Physiology— What's Happening?

SOME THINGS YOU can talk about forever, but until you've actually done them, you'll never really know what they are like. This applies to aerobatics. The combined sensations are unlike those encountered in any other human activity and must be experienced to be appreciated. Through the process of evolution, nature has provided man with a superbly well-adapted body for bipedal locomotion in one G, but she never seemed to have had aerobatic flying in mind. This is not to say that average healthy men and women cannot survive and even enjoy aerobatics—they can. However, aerobatics poses conditions alien to humans and the limits must be recognized. In this chapter, we shall discuss the physiology of aerobatics. A knowledge of this physiology should reduce your apprehension and distraction when you first encounter symptoms. In many areas, understanding the causes and effects of certain symptoms will allow the pilot and his passenger to take preventive steps to lessen the effect. Such preventive steps can safely extend the

142

range of human experience. The aerobatic aircraft of today is extremely strong and has the capability to perform to the limits set by the pilot's physiology. The observation of Louis Blériot, first man to fly across the English Channel, remains true after three-fourths of a century of flight:

> "It is not the resistance of matter which limits the aerobatic performance of the artificial bird [the airplane], but the physiological resistance of man, who is the bird's brain."

We would not want the situation to be otherwise. The alternative would be to have machines that could easily be pulled apart. However, since man is the limiting link in the chain, the pilot needs to understand his own limits and work within them.

THE INNER EAR, ORIENTATION AND MOTION SICKNESS

Our orientation in space is determined by sight, pressures on various parts of our bodies and, most important, our inner ear. In putting the inner ear at the top of the list, nature has rendered the best compromise, for this organ allows us to walk in total darkness to pursue or to avoid pursuit. What's best for an evolving, large-brained mammal, however, isn't necessarily best for the aerobatic pilot, so he needs to use all of the information available.

The most useful source of orientation information in aerobatics comes from vision. The pilot is strapped to his machine and only senses the G forces and accelerations, while his eyes give a complete summary. Often the loudest signal, from the inner ear, will be in conflict with what the other signals are saying and this conflict of signals can produce disorientation at both the conscious level ("I'm lost") and the unconscious level ("I'm sick").

The inner ear can be viewed as a fluid-filled cavity. Hairlike sensors located all around the cavity tell where the fluid is located, thereby signalling head position to the brain. When you are sitting erect, for example, the fluid pushes on the bottom and the brain reads this signal as being upright. If you are seated in an accelerating aircraft, the fluid pushes on the rear side of the cavity and the brain says that you're accelerating; opposite signals come through during deceleration. When the acceleration stops and the speed is constant, the fluid becomes stationary again and the brain thinks you're stationary unless you look out the window. Then, a brief disorientation occurs, followed by the rebalancing of the visual information and the inner ear information by that remarkable reprogrammable computer, the human brain.

If you are rotating, the fluid moves to the opposite side and tells the brain that you're spinning. This signal continues even if the rotation speed is constant. However, if you abruptly stop, the fluid can slosh to the other side and make you think that you've begun spinning in the opposite direction. The stagger following a rapid merry-go-round ride results from such signal switching.

Since the pilot's head is riding with the airplane but the inner ear fluid is free to move about, it is possible to receive conflicting signals from the eyes and the inner ears. Experience in this situation allows the conflicting signals to be sorted out and the correct diagnosis to be made.

It is this ability of the brain to learn from previous experience that makes aerobatics physiologically easier each time they are flown. The adaptive capabilities of the human brain and body are enormous, but they take time. For this reason, aerobatics should be introduced at an acceptable rate. If this caution is not observed, the result is disorientation, nausea and air sickness; the learning process comes to a rapid stop and you may find yourself with your head in an airsickness bag—if you're quick enough. Doctors still do not understand why the stomach being emptied should be a reaction to disorientation but it is, and you should be prepared for the worst just in case.

Susceptibility to motion sickness is difficult to predict. Almost anyone can be made sick, given extreme stimuli, but in moderate situations individual responses can vary enormously. Military training studies have shown that 6 percent of all student pilots were airsick on their first flights and about 14 percent were airsick on at least one of their early flights. The fact that the body accommodates to these new circumstances is reflected in the fact that on their tenth flights only 1 percent of the student pilots were airsick.

Motion sickness can strike anyone; motivation will not stave it off, although motivation can increase the level of acceptance. Both Lord Nelson and Charles Darwin were highly susceptible to *mal de mer,* but their strong motivation allowed them to persevere on their sea voyages. That any creature can be brought down by this malady is illustrated by the authenticated case of fish being transported by ship becoming seasick! So don't be so certain that your big muscles and machismo will exempt you from suffering.

The important thing is that, given enough time and a moderate pace of exposure, everyone can accommodate to the disorientations produced by aerobactics. Short periods of aerobatics are best for the start. Moreover, the novice should do as much of the flying himself as he can, for he then has the help of the feedback signals coming from the feel of the controls. But even the most experienced pilot runs the risk of disorientation if he flies with an inner ear infection, which can accompany a head cold, because then the usual sensors are not working.

THE MIDDLE EAR AND PRESSURE CHANGES

The earth's atmosphere is a self-supporting ocean of air. At the bottom the density and pressure are greatest; as we go to higher altitudes air thins out rapidly. At sea level the atmospheric pressure is about 760 mm of mercury, and this pressure decreases about 3 percent for each rise of 1000 feet.

The middle ear is that portion which lies between the eardrum (tympanic membrane) and the inner ear, where the sound sensors are located. The air pressure inside the middle ear is kept at equilibrium with the outside atmosphere by means of a narrow tube (the eustachian tube) connected to the nasal cavity. When air flows freely through the eustachian tube everything is fine, but when the tube is blocked, one can experience discomfort or even intense pain.

As a pilot rises in altitude, the outside air pressure decreases and the air inside the middle ear expands. When the altitude changes by 500 feet the extra air pressure will push its way out of the eustachian tube, with a click or pop sound if the tube is slightly blocked. This automatic clearing of the pressure usually proceeds smoothly, aided by motion of the jaw through chewing action or yawning.

Coming down is a different matter. The eustachian tube is constructed like a one-way valve and the higher air pressure on the outside has to force its way in. During a slow descent accompanied by jaw movement (which tugs the one-way valve open) the pressures equalize. In the event that the ears don't "keep up" with the pressure, closing the mouth and blowing against the pinched nostrils (the Valsalva maneuver) will often add enough additional pressure to equalize the pressure with a loud noise. If the pressure difference goes beyond that for about 2700 feet of altitude, then the eustachian tubes will be thoroughly stopped and the only relief lies in climbing back up to a lower pressure and starting over. This extra pressure may cause severe pain, deafness and, possibly, mild vertigo. When the pressure difference exceeds that for 3300 feet, there is the possibility of the eardrum rupturing, with accompanying vertigo and nausea.

Obviously, such extreme situations are infrequent but the potential is always there, especially if you are flying with a sore throat or with nasal congestion. If you have trouble clearing your ears on the way up, this is a sure sign of a problem and one that should be heeded.

The Valsalva maneuver is a last-resort action; if simple motion of the jaw does not suffice, you shouldn't be flying on such a day. Nose drops and sprays can be effective, especially if used before the flight; however, once their effect has worn off, the nasal passages will become even more blocked.

Because of the potential for debilitating vertigo, the wisest course is to avoid aerobatics altogether if you have a head cold. In the case of a sore throat, there is the potential for a "pinched" ear; therefore, rapid and large changes of altitude should be avoided.

POSITIVE G FORCES

The G forces caused by change of direction are an integral part of aerobatics and are present day after day. The pilot should definitely understand them. Large positive G forces produce a heaviness and flirting with loss of vision or even loss of consciousness. Large negative G forces are simply uncomfortable and painful. The physiological bases for these symptoms are quite different and need to be understood, for this understanding should help you take appropriate preventative actions.

G forces relate most importantly to blood supply and its distribution in the body. In order to understand this, we need to understand some elements of the human anatomy. The accompanying figure illustrates the basic elements that play a role

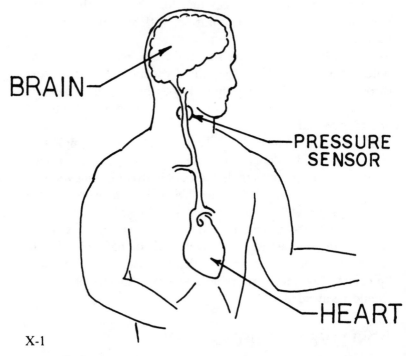

BRAIN

PRESSURE
SENSOR

HEART

X-1

The most important parts of the human body—as far as G forces are concerned—are the heart, the pressure sensors in the arteries supplying blood to the brain and the brain itself.

in G forces. The heart pumps blood to all parts of the body but one-fourth of the supply goes to the head, where it supplies the brain. Below the heart is the large volume of the body cavity and the largest artery, the aorta. Connected about this system are various pressure sensors that have been preprogrammed to respond to changes as necessary for hunt, pursuit and escape, which doesn't mean that our bodies are also made for aerobatic

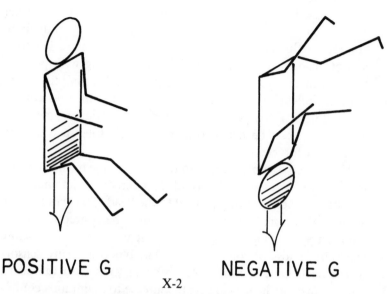

POSITIVE G   NEGATIVE G

X-2

Large positive G forces pool the blood in the lower part of the body and the legs, producing blackout. Large negative G forces try to push the blood into the head, producing extreme discomfort.

flying. Nevertheless, they're all that is available and we will have to make do for the present.

Positive G forces are those in which the pull on our body is in the usual downward sense. In a simplified sequence, let's see how increasingly large positive G forces act on the relaxed pilot or passenger. We are accustomed to one G; except when swimming or jumping, this is what we normally experience. At two G's the arms and legs definitely feel heavy as they are held extended to control the airplane. At three G's the entire body feels the load and the skin of the face may feel as though it is sagging down (it is). At four G's the muscular symptoms are all increased, and the pilot may suffer a loss of vision, either experiencing tunnel vision or seeing everything uniformly faint. Sometimes this is followed by "seeing stars." At five G's total loss of vision will often occur (blackout), along with possible loss of consciousness. This discussion is highly simplified, but it does indicate the entire gamut of symptoms that can be encountered. Fortunately, there are automatic and artificial actions that can be taken to increase one's tolerance to high positive G forces.

The failure of blood supply to the brain is due to the fact that more blood pressure is needed to overcome the increased weight of the blood being pushed to the head. The eyes have an additional internal pressure which must be overcome by the blood supply. This is why vision impairment occurs before blackout or loss of consciousness. The blood pressure sensors in the neck have a positive feedback relation with the heart, which cause the heartbeat rate to increase to maintain a continuous flow of blood to the brain. This change of heartbeat takes about five seconds to take effect and if the onset of the G forces is very rapid, a temporary loss of blood supply can occur. This means that the rate of onset of the G forces is important, as is the duration. The schematic diagram illustrates the relation between G forces, duration and the rate at which the G forces are encountered. Very short loads are unimportant, since there is a reservoir of oxygen-rich blood in the head which is enough for about five seconds. Rapid loads can produce blackout before the heartbeat rate increases, but after about five seconds it usually catches up. Tolerance to G loads goes down with very long exposures as the compensation mechanisms fail.

You can take several actions to reduce the effects of high positive G forces. The principal two actions available to the ordinary aerobatic pilot can increase his tolerance by about 2.4

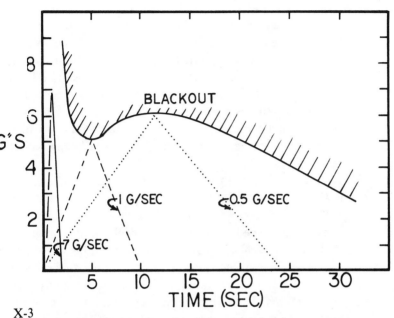

X-3

Different G forces can be tolerated for different lengths of time. Above the line, in the region marked BLACKOUT, *the average pilot will black out. If the G forces come on and are removed rapidly (7 G/second), then the tolerance is high because the blood reservoir in the head takes care of it. A slow rate of onset (0.5 G/second) gives the heart time to adjust while an intermediate rate (1 G/second) gives the lowest tolerance. (After a diagram by Gauer and Zuidema)*

G's, which makes a big difference in the ability to fly a high-performance aerobatic sequence. The simplest action is to tighten the abdominal muscles and upper leg *prior* to onset of the G forces. This action prevents pooling of blood in the body cavity and makes it available for transport to the head. A second action is to exhale slowly through a partially closed throat. One must be careful not to close the throat entirely, for this will act to reduce the tolerance to G forces. The best rule of thumb is, if the exhalation is noisy, then it is helping. World War II pilots were often trained to scream or shout, which simply isn't necessary. For sustained G forces, one should keep the lower muscles tight and continue the forced exhalation, taking short breaths as necessary. This procedure is usually referred to as the M-1 maneuver and needs to become an automatic response by the aerobatic pilot whenever he begins to feel positive G forces.

It is this anticipation of the results of G forces that allows the experienced aerobatic pilot to avoid the vision losses that can accompany the higher G forces. If the pilot's physical state is temporarily diminished by lack of physical conditioning, illness, or the residual effects of alcohol or tobacco, his safe range of tolerance will be reduced. This means that he can find himself blacked out or unconscious doing maneuvers that usually produce no symptoms. The natural tendency upon losing vision is to relax the back pressure that is producing the G forces. Visual effects disappear within seconds as the G force is relaxed. If actual loss of consciousness occurs, the situation is much more serious. Once the blackout has happened, it will last for about fifteen seconds, followed by a few seconds of disorientation. The loss of those twenty seconds can be very serious, especially at low altitude. An aircraft traveling at 60 miles per hour downward is losing altitude at the rate of 88 feet per second; not much time is left for recovery after a loss of consciousness at 1500 feet while finishing off a Hammerhead.

A word is appropriate here about physical conditioning. Being in superb physical condition cannot hurt, but it is probably sufficient to be in good condition. Back and stomach muscle condition is quite important and can be attained through an appropriate set of sit-up and back-bending exercises. The back muscles protect your back from the enormous loads that are imposed at high G forces. Strong stomach muscles can prevent the pooling of blood in the abdomen, which produces blackouts. Arm and wrist strength helps, but there are some small and highly successful women pilots who are proof that this is not a paramount requirement. Cardiovascular health is probably the major consideration and the best way to maintain this is through regular and extended exercise, such as running. If you look at a cross section of Unlimited Category aerobatic pilots, you certainly will find a few carrying some extra weight; but as a group, they can be best described as vigorous and healthy. If you're interested in aerobatics, get in shape.

NEGATIVE G FORCES

Negative G forces are those directed upward, toward the head of the seated pilot (figure X-2). Although they need to be handled with caution, early alarming reports of physiologists were undoubtedly inaccurate.

At the onset of negative G forces the sensations are much like those found in standing on one's head (minus one G), with a feeling of discomfort and fullness in the face. At higher negative G forces, discomfort is replaced with pain, fullness is replaced with distortion, occasionally producing broken blood vessels around the eyes. Sinus congestion and bleeding may be encountered. In the case of positive G forces, blackout is the limiting condition. In the negative G forces, there is a continuum of symptoms, without a natural cessation.

Discomfort arises from the forcing of blood into the head and the increase of blood pressure there as the negative G forces increase. Since the brain is surrounded by fluid in a closed box (the skull), the tissues of the brain come into balance with the extra pressure and little danger of bleeding is present. Early "destructive" tests on laboratory animals indicate that their collapse at negative G forces greater than minus ten were not the result of brain damage. Extended tests at negative G's by physiologists indicate no long-term effects of even repeated exposures.

The disturbing aspect of flying with negative G's is the action of the heart. The pressure sensors that detected low blood supply and increased the heart rate during positive G forces now do the opposite. An extraordinarily high blood pressure is sensed and the heart is told to slow. The average heartbeat rate drops by about 40 percent at minus three G's and is characterized by groups of beats followed by stoppages of several seconds. The healthy human heart is remarkably resilient, but because of the stresses negative G aerobatics is an activity one needs to enter with an unquestioned clean bill of health.

There have been some reports of a redout occurring at high negative G forces. However, there are no authenticated cases from studies of centrifuge volunteers and controlled studies of aerobatic pilots. Perhaps the rare true case of redout arises from the lower eyelid being pulled over the eye, although this explanation does not seem satisfactory since the corresponding phenomenon is not found at high positive G levels.

This chapter has made aerobatic flying sound like entering a torture chamber. To the contrary, flying aerobatics is physically challenging, stimulating and just plain fun. It is serious fun, however, and must be approached with one's eyes wide open and a willingness to prepare oneself physically. If you know the causes of the sensations you experience, they become less threatening. The pilot is left free to fly within his own safe range of operation.

11
Organizations—
Assistance

PEOPLE WITH COMMON INTERESTS, experiences and needs tend to draw together and aerobatics is no exception. Since the late 1960s there has been a rapid growth in membership of organizations that have brought aerobatic flying to many thousands of pilots and enthusiasts. It's hardly surprising that such organizations come into existence, for many of us are interested in extending the realm of flight, and the fastest progress lies in building on the experience of others.

There is much wisdom in the saying of George Santayana that "those who cannot remember the past are condemned to repeat it." We cannot hope to remember the unsuccessful trials that have been done before if we don't first learn about them. The national organizations are an excellent way to learn what has happened before and how to begin building from that foundation. The subject is developing so rapidly that one person alone cannot really stay abreast of what is happening.

These organizations serve two major functions: encouraging

155

and serving the aerobatic flying community and arranging for aerobatic competitions. In addition, they explain and represent the aerobatic community in dealings with the government. They do these jobs very well.

There are two major aerobatic organizations: the Aerobatic Club of America and the International Aerobatic Club. They have complementary roles and both play an important part in American aerobatics.

THE AEROBATIC CLUB OF AMERICA

The Aerobatic Club of America (ACA) was organized in 1964 to administer the sport of aerobatics in the United States. It was created in response to a particular set of needs—to conduct American sport aerobatics in a way consistent with international rules, to field a United States aerobatic team in international competition and to name a national champion. World competition was begun in 1960 under the aegis of the Fédération Aeronautique Internationale (FAI), which is the worldwide governing body in the field of records and sport aviation. This body designates one aero club in each nation to carry out the FAI's functions. Within the United States, this organization is the National Aeronautic Association (NAA). Within its broad charter, the NAA appointed the ACA to administer the sport of aerobatics from 1969 to 1982. This genealogy shows not only the ACA's pedigree but also indicates what its primary emphasis has been. In its early years it sanctioned the contest that chose the National Champions and selected the United States team. Later, as the International Aerobatic Club developed additional categories of competition, the ACA began naming National Champions in each of those categories.

In 1982 the NAA recognized the larger and more vigorous organization of the International Aerobatic Club (IAC) and gave the IAC authority for administering aerobatics in the United States. The ACA is now in the process of dissolving its organization.

THE INTERNATIONAL AEROBATIC CLUB

The primary purpose of the IAC is to promote safe aerobatic flying and to make it possible for a large portion of the aviation community to participate in aerobatics. The IAC was formed in 1970 as a division of the Experimental Aircraft Association (EAA). Even though it started small, it is rapidly growing, with more than 3700 members and 40 active local chapters. It is a grass-roots organization with a strong emphasis on aerobatics at all levels, including the most elementary. It sponsors activities within geographic and financial reach of almost all pilots in the United States and has a growing number of members from other nations. The IAC is led by an elected set of officers and a board of directors, who conduct the business of the organization. On a local basis, there are the chapters, which are chartered, self-governing, groups of members.

Since the IAC is a division of the EAA, a word about the parent organization is appropriate. The EAA was formed in 1953 in Milwaukee as a small organization of sport aviation enthusiasts who shared an interest in construction of custom-built (Experimental category) aircraft. From these simple beginnings, it has grown to include more than 90,000 members and 700 chapters, spread across all 50 states and over 100 foreign countries. Its emphasis remains on custom-built aircraft but in addition to the IAC, it has added three other divisions for related special-interest groups, the Antique and Classic Division, the Warbirds of America, and the Ultralight Association. The EAA, the largest sport aviation organization in the world, seeks to educate the public about sport aviation and to protect the interests of the sport.

The IAC provides many services to its members. The most visible service is the monthly magazine *Sport Aerobatics,* which thoroughly covers the aerobatic scene, including articles on flying contests, maintenance of aerobatic aircraft, how-to-do and chapter activities. Other services, the direct interaction with the FAA, for example, are less visible. This role has been an important one, for it has created a basically positive attitude toward organized aerobatics on the part of the federal agency. The IAC has earned this position, for the emphasis has always been on safety and its record is excellent.

Information about the IAC, aerobatics, and aerobatic flight schools can be obtained by writing: International Aerobatic

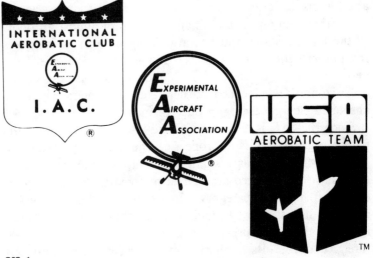

XI-1

The International Aerobatic Club operates as a division of the Experimental Aircraft Association. The United States Aerobatic Foundation was recently begun to support the United States team in world competitions.

Club, Wittman Airport, Oshkosh, WI 54903-2591, or calling 414-426-4800.

UNITED STATES AEROBATIC FOUNDATION

When the IAC was charged by NAA with administering aerobatics in the United States, it had a fundamental problem. IAC is the *International* Aerobatic Club and includes an important group of members who are from countries other than the United States of America. The problem was that one of the new administrative functions was to select and field a United States team for the World Aerobatic Championships. This problem was resolved by creating a new, separate organization, the United States Aerobatic Foundation (the Foundation). The function of the Foundation is to field and support the United States aerobatic team at the biennial World Championships, with no resources of the IAC being used for this purpose. This is a formidable task, because the flying team can be as large as five men and five women, and requires a comparably sized support staff of team leaders, trainers, judges, mechanics, interpreters, doctors, etc. Since the World contest is usually held abroad (it has been in the United States only once, in 1980), planes, pilots, and other team members must be transported to Europe and then supported in the field during not only the contest but also for the practice period beforehand. Recognizing this, it is not surprising that a primary task of the Foundation is fund-raising. The United States team gets no financial support from its government, so you and I are the sources of support.

IAC ACTIVITIES

The IAC becomes most visible through its activities. These include contests, achievement awards, judges' schools and chapter activities. (Contests will be discussed in chapter 13.) Achievement awards are citations earned by individual pilots as measures of their proficiency in flying aerobatics, judged on uniform national standards. There are five categories, of increasing difficulty. In each category there is a list of the types of maneuvers that must be done. The exact maneuver selected is up to the pilot. Table 3 lists the requirements for each category: Basic, Sportsman, Intermediate, Advanced and Unlimited. A pilot earning all of these awards qualifies for an ALL FIVE patch. Each maneuver can be done separately, even on different flights and days. They can be done at any altitude above certain minimums as long as the judge can clearly see the maneuver. The maneuvers must be flown in front of a judge accredited by the IAC and with a quality indicated by a score of 5 on the 0-10 scale used in judging (chapter 12). If you miss reaching this quality of performance, you can try the maneuver over on another day, until the list is complete.

Since these maneuvers can be done one at a time, altitude can be traded for entry speed and even low-power aircraft can be used in pursuing the tougher categories, although a certain point is reached at which inverted fuel systems become a must. Since any IAC member is free to work on these at any time, the pursuit of achievement awards is essentially continuous.

The more difficult four categories can be earned "With Stars" by flying in competition. In this case, all of the normal contest rules are used and a score of 5 or better must be earned from all five judges on all maneuvers on all flights in that contest. The specific maneuvers to be flown are those designated for the contest, rather than the list for the starless awards (Smooth Patches). Since the awards "With Stars" demand doing the maneuvers back-to-back and not lapsing badly on even one, "Achievement Awards With Stars" are much more difficult to earn. A pilot who earns all of the Smooth Patch and "With Stars" awards qualifies for a special ALL NINE patch. This is

ACHIEVEMENT AWARDS
(REQUIRED MANEUVERS)

BASIC	SPORTSMAN	INTERMEDIATE	ADVANCED	UNLIMITED
Loop	Loop	Square Loop	Square Loop	Hammerhead with inverted entry
Spin (one turn)	Spin (one turn)	Spin (one turn)	Spin (one turn)	Inverted Spin (one turn)
Roll (any type)	Immelmann	Immelmann	Immelmann	360° rolling circle with rolls to the outside (number optional)
	Half Cuban	Half Cuban	Half Cuban	Tailside
	Snap Roll	Diving Snap Roll on 45° line	Snap Roll on climbing or diving 45°line	Cuban Eight (double outside)
	Slow Roll	Slow Roll on 45° climbing line	Eight Point Roll	Outside Snap Roll
	Barrel Roll	Super Slow Roll	Super Slow Roll	Vertical Diving Snap Roll
	Hammerhead	Four Point Roll	Reverse Half Cuban	Eight Point Roll
	Reverse Half Cuban	Hammerhead with quarter rolls up and down	Outside Loop	Outside Loop
		Reverse Half Cuban	English Bunt	Vertical Roll (at least 180°)
			Layout Eight	Eight Sided Loop
			360° rolling circle (number of rolls optional)	
			Vertical Half Roll with pushover	

part of the endless challenge of aerobatics and here the competition is against oneself and no one else. As of April 1983, more than 2800 achievement awards have been issued, 25 pilots receiving the ALL NINE patch.

Judges' schools are held at a number of locations throughout the United States every year. Their purpose is to train people interested in judging at contests and for the achievement awards. These schools use standardized grading criteria and are the basis for uniform judging at all IAC activities. Usually they are composed of two parts, a lecture by an experienced judge, using many visual aids, and flight demonstrations of well and poorly executed maneuvers. A programmed learning curriculum has recently been developed.

Chapter activities vary widely in content and frequency. Some chapters meet monthly, others upon demand. Some have regular lectures, teaching the neophyte the basics of aerobatics. Many host regular weekend flying events in which everyone judges everyone else. Often these weekend events are used to pursue achievement awards. Perhaps the most ambitious undertaking of a chapter is the sponsoring of a contest. With the exception of the IAC championships and the nationals, all contests are sponsored by chapters.

There are about 30 regional contests sponsored by the IAC each year, usually during the warm weather months. These contests range from small affairs of local interest to regional events that draw pilots from many states. These are usually relaxed events reflecting the color and flavor of the area. If you examine the calendar of events published in *Sport Aerobatics,* you'll probably find at least one contest each year near you.

The National Championship contest is usually held in the South in the autumn. Frequently, the site has been in Texas, where the autumn weather permits one to schedule open cockpit flying. The time of year also allows the competitors to take advantage of the experience from a full season of competition on the IAC circuit. It is an intense competition, for this is the only chance for a National Championship. Since the world championship is usually scheduled for alternate years, the top unlimited pilots from the National Championship have the opportunity to represent the United States every other year. Membership on the United States team can be and has been the stepping stone to becoming World Champion. It is no wonder that this contest is taken very seriously.

There is an aerobatic organization for almost any serious enthusiast. The armchair types and the unlimited competitors and everyone in between can find some benefit in belonging to the IAC.

12
Evaluating Maneuvers— How Good Is Good?

JUDGING IS AS IMPORTANT as flying in today's American aerobatic scene. It is the factor that sets precision aerobatics apart as a true art, one with well-defined criteria that are the same throughout the country. It is an activity pursued by persons from a variety of backgrounds, both pilots and non-pilots. It is sometimes argued that only someone who has been there can accurately judge aerobatics, but this is hardly the case, for such pilots have certain prejudices based on whether or not a particular maneuver is difficult for them. Many of the best judges in the United States today are not active aerobatic pilots. They do not vicariously "feel" the loads the pilot is feeling and are therefore free to evaluate the maneuvers on the basis of simple, well-defined criteria. This is a low-cost way of participating in a somewhat expensive sport, for there is no hangar rent to be paid nor are there bad cylinders to be overhauled. What does it take to be a judge? A willingness to study the criteria, apprentice oneself for a period of "on-the-job training" and consistent

164

application of objective standards of performance, regardless of the fame of the pilot or the maneuvers he has just done.

If you are more interested in flying than judging, it is still essential that you understand the methods and criteria of judging, for these are the rules of the game. Having these rules makes the activity uniform and gives a continuous challenge to the aerobatic pilot. They are rules made by pilots for pilots and are natural ways of flying aircraft in aerobatics.

Taken apart, element by element, aerobatic flying can be done perfectly. A line can be straight or an angle exact, a roll rate constant or a spin stopped exactly on the right heading. If the individual elements can be done perfectly, then there is the potential that whole maneuvers can be done without error and given that, why not entire sequences? It is this taste of perfection in small bites that attracts us in aerobatics, even if the goal seems to recede almost as fast as we pursue it. Grading ourselves and grading others gives the opportunity to see how close we are to that Aerobatic nirvana.

BASIC PRINCIPLES OF JUDGING MANEUVERS

The basic principles applied in judging are the same for both the IAC and CIVA. They assume that a maneuver is being flown perfectly until something is seen to be wrong (innocent until proved guilty, if you will) and that scoring should be unambiguous and quantitative. These goals are approached very closely and it is that slight gap at the end that demands the judgment in judging. Experience is necessary for acquiring the ability to make the necessary judgments and even the quantitative responses. This is why all aerobatic groups require some actual field experience. The more important levels of competition require more experience.

Scoring of maneuvers always begins with a score of 10 and can be reduced by increments of 0.5 right down to 0 on the basis of observed errors. This means that everyone starts with a 10.0 and, through errors, works his way down. Since there are quantitative standards for the amounts to be deducted for errors in each element of a maneuver, enough mistakes can quickly bring a score down to 0, but still be a recognizable example of that maneuver. This is essential to understand. A score of 0 does not mean the maneuver is unrecognizable; it simply means that enough errors were found to reduce the score by 10. Some people may jump to the conclusion that 0 is terrible, 5 is fair and 10 is perfect, but this is not true. Ten *is* perfect, but intermediate scores are based on individual subtractions. For example, a complex maneuver like a Horizontal Eight has at least eight elements that are easily judged; and losing only a little more than one point on each element would bring a pilot down to 0, even though the basic maneuver didn't look all that bad. This is why the more complex maneuvers have higher K (difficulty) factors and if you want to score well, you'd better stick with the simpler maneuvers.

Maneuvers are judged one by one and a pilot may do one maneuver beautifully then almost spin out of the next. The only exception to this one-at-a-time rule is for the Four Minute Program flown by Unlimited pilots. The judging rules there differ significantly and will be discussed later in Chapter XIII. The judge must be able to erase his memory after each maneuver has been scored, so that the "halo" effect doesn't cause him to score high all the maneuvers in a flight while there were one or two bad ones sprinkled in. The opposite effect can also occur and must be avoided just as conscientiously. The pace of flying can be very fast, especially in the higher categories with their complex maneuvers. The judge must be able to give his score quickly, then immediately devote all his attention to the next maneuver.

ELEMENTS OF MANEUVERS

Each maneuver is judged by the quality of its elements, and wherever possible quantitative guidelines have been established. There are relatively few elements and they form the basis of the score. Maneuvers can be composed of Attitude, Headings, Banks, Lines (track), Roll, Autorotations, Curves, Hesitations, Pivots and Altitude.

Attitude, Heading, Lines and Bank are graded by the 5° rule. That is, for each 5° off the desired angle you subtract 1.0 from the score. If you see an error of less than 5°, you can still take off 0.5 point. This means that if, in the performance of an otherwise perfect Hammerhead, on the down line the aircraft had an attitude of 75° instead of 90°, then 3 (three increments of 5° off) points would be subtracted. That maneuver would be given a score of 7. Similarly, if it had been flown 70° on the way up and 87° on the way down, then 4 would be taken off for the first error and 0.5 for the second error and the score would be 5.5. The same type of rule applies to projected Lines, Headings and Banks. All of these are applied to one maneuver, so you can see how much flying skill is needed to hold on to that starting score of 10. All these elements are graded with respect to the ideal with the exception of the Bank used in turns, which must be a *minimum* of 60°, with 1 point subtracted for each 5° below that, but no penalty assessed for bank angles above 60°.

The other elements listed are scored more qualitatively. Roll can be at any rate but it must be constant. Using this criteria eliminates any advantage of one airplane over another. Since roll rate can vary with airspeed, this is something to which the judge and the pilot must be alert. The only time constraint on any roll is the Super Slow Roll, which must take a minimum of 15 seconds for one full rotation. Taking less than 15 seconds means by definition that a Roll and not a Super Slow Roll was flown and a score of 0 would be given. The faster the roll rate,

THE 5° RULE

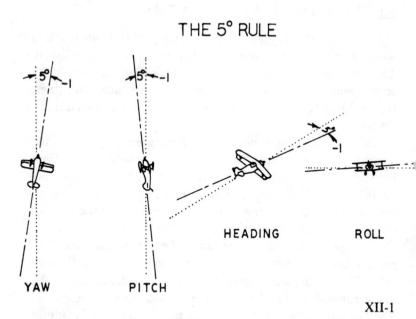

YAW PITCH HEADING ROLL

XII-1

The 5° rule is basic to judging all aerobatic maneuvers. Each deviation of 5° from the desired orientation results in subtraction of one point from the score for that maneuver.

the less likely it is for the rate to vary and it is hardly any wonder that no one seems to voluntarily fly Super Slow Rolls for score. Varying the roll rate slightly may subtract as little as 0.5 while varying it a lot may cost the pilot as much as 2.0.

Autorotation is either there or it isn't. In the Spins and the Snap Rolls, one looks for the smooth motion at a high angle of attack. It is possible to "cheat" on these maneuvers by using the ailerons at entry and exit, especially at the start of a Spin when the pilot wants to spin in one direction and not the other. Be alert to this and take off a point if you see it happen. Of course, if the autorotation never really occurs, the maneuver must be given a 0. A final common error is to underrotate on either the Spin or Snap and to use the ailerons to continue the Roll until the wings are level or the right heading is assumed. The 5° rule applies here also. It will be more obvious if the pilot overrotates, and the same 5° rule applies.

Curves are encountered in looping and turning maneuvers. In the Loop the radius does not matter; what we are looking for is that the radius be constant. A perfect Loop made at high speed and power describing an enormous area may be spectacular, but it is worth the same 10 points as a perfectly round Loop done at a small radius. How much is subtracted for non-roundness (in constant radius) varies qualitatively with the amount. A Loop done at the same entry and exit altitudes and good heading control, but badly out of round may score as low as 3 or 4 and another in which the pilot pinches the five-eighths' region only slightly may be a 9. One needs to be especially alert to roundness in the maneuvers that involve only partial loops, since there is usually a tendency to pinch (tighten the Loop) or float (enlarge the Loop) just before starting the connecting line. In the horizontal turn one looks for constant Bank Angle but in the Rolling Turns this translates to a constant rate of turn.

Hesitations occur during the Hesitation Rolls and the Family 9 maneuvers. In the Hesitation Rolls consistency is again the key, for the pauses can be of any length, as long as they are well defined and constant. If there is only one point (pause), there is no problem, and this can occur in a Half Four Point Roll. In the case of multiple points, the first one should set the pattern for the rest. It is common to see the pauses become shorter and shorter as the roll continues, especially in the 8 and 16 Point Rolls. Hesitations also play a role in the Family 9 maneuvers, such as the Immelmann, Split S and Fishhooks. In the Immelmann, the Half Loop portion is completed and the inverted horizontal position is held only long enough to establish recognition of the horizontal, then the Half Roll is begun. Here we are looking for the pilot to just "kiss" the line, then immediately start to roll. If the inverted line is projected, then the maneuver should be downgraded. The same is true for the Split S, in which the inverted position after the Half Roll is held just momentarily before the pull through is begun. The final example of "kissing" lines is the Fishhooks. These are maneuvers in which a descending 45° line is followed by a three-eighths loop, a brief vertical line and then a return to the original level flight track. The vertical line is, again, just long enough to establish the correct attitude, immediately followed by a push to level flight.

The pivot occurs in the Hammerhead. It is important that the aircraft pivots and does not fly around the top. If the maneuver is started prematurely, the aircraft will move to the side as it comes over the top; started too late, the aircraft will do a form of slide. What the judge looks for is upward motion almost stopped and a pivot within the wingspan of the aircraft. A common error is for the pivot to not be in the same plane; this is commonly called torque, although we saw before that the outside wing producing more lift was the principal culprit.

A final element and one that is easy to judge is altitude. Loops and some of the eights require big altitude changes, but are intended to end at the same altitude as the entry. The wise judge usually holds up a pencil or some mark to record the entry altitude, which makes it possible to judge altitudes to within a small margin even from several thousand feet. Other maneuvers, such as the Roll and Turn, are to be done at constant altitude. Some maneuvers simply require that the first and last portions be done at constant altitude, but these elements are important nonetheless. It is most common to see altitude changes at the entry to spins, when the airspeed is changing rapidly. Again, the reference mark is an accurate and unforgiving aid.

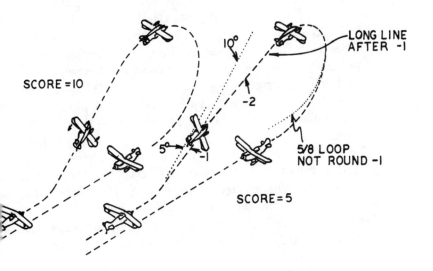

SCORE = 10

10°

LONG LINE
AFTER -1

-2

5°

-1

5/8 LOOP
NOT ROUND -1

SCORE = 5

MANEUVER 9.2.1.2.1

XII-2

The perfectly flown Reverse Half Cuban shown on the left keeps the score of 10 that it was given at the start. The imperfect maneuver shown on the right lost points for heading, track errors, unequal line lengths and the looping portion not being round.

SCORING MANEUVERS

Judging involves much, much more than the above comments, but these should cover most situations, especially in the early stages of flying aerobatics. Let's apply these principles to two illustrative maneuvers, a Reverse Half Cuban (figure XII-2) and a Hammerhead (figure XII-3).

The Reverse Half Cuban started very nicely but the pilot was 5° off heading after the one-eighth Loop (−1), correcting for this gradually during the rest of the maneuver. After setting the line and rolling upright he was quite shallow (35°, −2) and drew the second line much too long (−1). Then he pinched the Loop in pulling down to the horizontal line (−1). Score for maneuver: 5.

The Hammerhead is flown with about the same general quality. In this case the pilot was below the vertical by 5° (−1) but then caught it and corrected on the way up. He flew over the top (−1), made a shorter vertical on the way down (−1) and tried to compensate by making a larger-radius Quarter Loop on the bottom (−0.5), but still ended up higher than where he started. Final score: 6.5.

Do this in real time, about every 15 to 20 seconds for three to eight minutes and you'll see that judging can be a fast-paced activity. The added distractions of glare from the sun, heat and an uncomfortable chair can only add to the challenge. Still, people come back to this job, for it is just as important as the flying. It is not altogether without reward, because judges always get trophies at contests, whereas most contestants don't. It requires attendance at a two-day judge's school (given many times a year at various spots around the country) and it does take homework, for there is a long open-book examination. In addition, one must satisfy an experience requirement. This sounds like a lot of work but it is worth it. It is fair to say that within organized aerobatics the best judges are as respected as the most successful pilots, and as a judge moves up through the ranks of Regional, National and International Judge he gets more recognition.

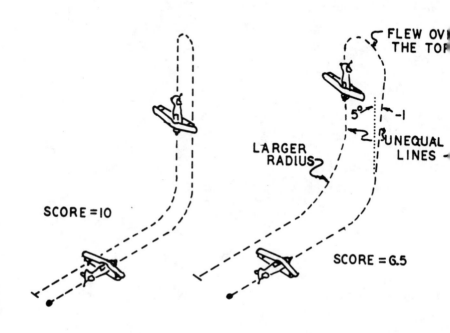

SCORE = 10

SCORE = 6.5

LARGER RADIUS

FLEW OV[ER] THE TOP

5°

UNEQUAL LINES

MANEUVER 5.1.1

XII-3

The Hammerhead is very easy to judge in terms of vertical attitude, timing of the pivot, line length, radius of Quarter Loops and altitudes.

13
Contest Flying – The Measure of Man and Machine

IN THIS CHAPTER, we'll talk about how an aerobatic contest is organized and what happens at one. The primary goal of an organized aerobatic contest is safety. It is a goal that is never compromised by its chairman. Vigilance is the key word, and vigilance is observed in the standards of the aircraft allowed to enter, in the qualifications of the pilots and in the way the flying is conducted.

CATEGORY FLYING

American aerobatic contests are organized around a category system developed by the IAC. It is a system based on the type and difficulty of the maneuvers in four different categories. Since the categories are defined by what flying is done in them, the system is left to sort itself out in terms of ability of the pilot and the capability of the aircraft. As we'll see, there is no way a 115-hp Citabria could compete in the most difficult category, even if piloted by last year's champion in that same category. Likewise, it would be impossible for a novice aerobatic pilot (with more money than flying experience) to buy an all-out competition machine and start anywhere but at the simplest categories. The system is similar to weight divisions in boxing, but without exact weight guidelines. A big, new heavyweight might only be well-matched in light weights at the start but would want to move up as he becomes more competitive. On the other hand, a welterweight is never going to beat a heavyweight, but it's still grand to be welterweight champion. The actual requirement is to be able to fly safely in a particular category and to be able to perform 60 percent of the maneuvers. There is a certain competitive element in us all, and few pilots move up in category unless they are not only safe, but also have a reasonable chance of winning.

The most popular category is Sportsman (about 45 percent of competitors). It has two flights, a Known Compulsory and a Free Program. The compulsory maneuvers are all selected from the Aresti Families that do not require sustained inverted flight or high power-to-weight ratios. As in all Known Compulsory flights, a standard sequence of maneuvers is set up for the year and is flown at each contest. Usually there are about ten maneuvers and a total difficulty value of about 140 K. The total K value allowed for the Free Program is adjusted each year to be the same as for that year's Known Compulsory, which allows the pilot to refly the same sequence if he desires. Since this category is the simplest in its demands on airplane and pilot, you will see a variety of airplanes in it, as well as many first-time competitors. Some pilots never move up from Sportsman because of their machines or the amount of aerobatic flying that they do, and the annual race is to see if the less experienced pilots in their high-performance machines can beat the "old pros" in their Clipped Wing Cubs.

The next category is Intermediate. The pilots fly three times, but different sequences each time. The first flight is also a

SPORTSMAN
K=130

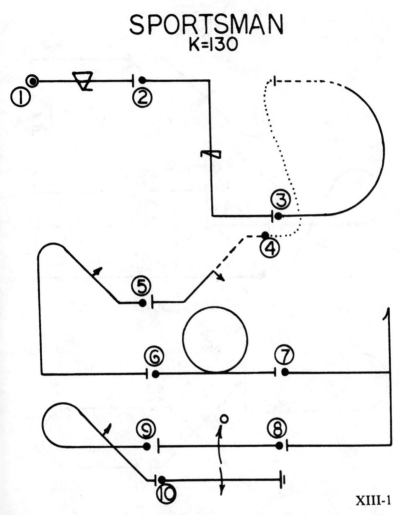

XIII-1

The Sportsman category sequence is the simplest competition flight. It does not require an inverted fuel and oil system and uses the most elementary maneuvers out of many families in the Aresti catalog.

INTERMEDIATE
K=202

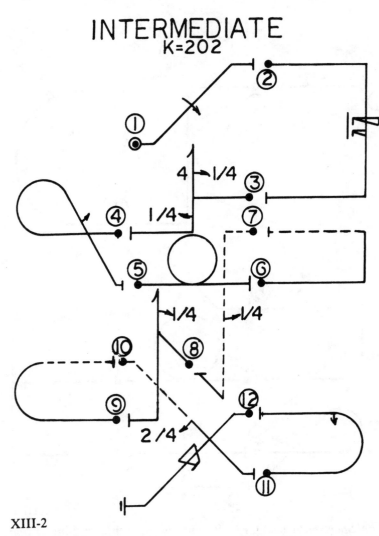

XIII-2

The Intermediate category sequence requires an aircraft with inverted fuel and oil systems because it involves sustained inverted flight. Some "frills" are seen on a few of the maneuvers.

Known Compulsory, but this one is composed of about 14 maneuvers and has a total difficulty of about 200 K. The second flight is a Free Program of no more than 20 maneuvers and no more than 250 K. In both flights, the average maneuvers will be more difficult and will involve sustained inverted flight, Quarter Rolls on Vertical Lines and even full rolls on 45° lines. The composition of the Free Program is left to the judgment of the pilot, constrained only by including certain types of maneuvers characteristic of that category. He must, however, declare the flight sequence beforehand and follow it as religiously as a Known Compulsory sequence. He cannot ad lib or pretend that he had really intended the third maneuver to be an Inverted Spin instead of the second half of a Square Loop. We'll discuss below how the Free Programs are composed.

The Unknown Compulsory is challenging to fly and fun to watch. The flight sequence is given to the pilots the evening before they are to fly and the first time they fly it is in front of the judges! It is the equivalent of a sight-reading test in a music contest. Since every pilot is flying the same sequence, the spectator and the spectating fellow competitor know what is to come next and watch for that fatal goof that means the pilot has lost his place on the sequence card or in the midst of the rush from one maneuver to the next has put in a Loop for a Half Cuban. It's a rare contest where someone doesn't come down with egg on his face. We've all had our turns at this part. About 30 percent of all competitors are flying in this category.

The Advanced category pilot is allowed three flights, the Known Compulsory (about 18 maneuvers and 350 K), the Free Program (no more than 20 maneuvers and 400 K) and an Unknown Compulsory (about 12 maneuvers and 250 K). All of the flights involve about one-fifth outside maneuvers, fractional vertical rolls, Rolling Turns to the inside and many compound maneuvers. About 15 percent of all competitors fly in the Advanced category.

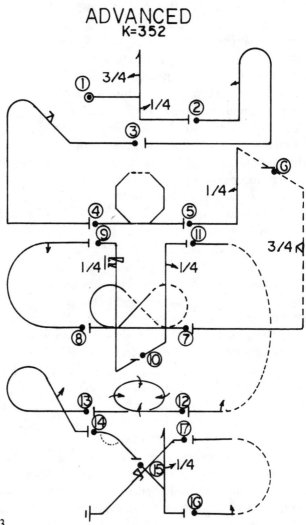

XIII-3

The Advanced category sequence is characterized by more and more complex maneuvers in addition to a sprinkling of outside maneuvers.

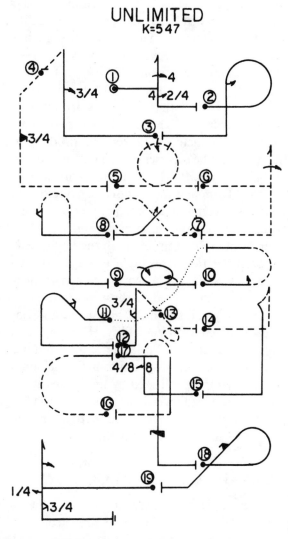

XIII-4

Almost anything goes in the Unlimited category sequence. There are numerous outside, vertical and compound maneuvers. At less than 20 seconds per maneuver, a lot happens—and quickly.

Unlimited category means just that. Almost anything in the Aresti Catalog of maneuvers is fair game and you'll see most of it at one time or another. There are four flights: a Known Compulsory (about 22 maneuvers and 450 K), a Free Program (no more than 23 maneuvers and 700 K), an Unknown Compulsory (about 15 maneuvers and 450 K) and a Four Minute Program. Almost half of the maneuvers are outside and full vertical rolls are common. The maneuvers are difficult and can be done down to 100 meters (328 feet) of altitude. Competitors in this category must be experienced, confident and possess high performance machines. It is from this category that the United States National Team and the National Champion are chosen. Only about 10 percent of all competitors are found in this category, and their commitment is *very* high.

The Four Minute Program found in the Unlimited category deserves special mention. This flight is judged as a total flight and not a simple sum of the scores of each maneuver. Any maneuver can be done, including those not in the Aresti Catalog. This is where you'll see the Torque Rolls and Lomcevaks. The flight is evaluated upon Versatility, Harmony and Rhythm, Originality, Execution and Positioning. Any number of maneuvers can be done, but programs usually include about 14. No sequence program is followed by the judges and what you get is what you see. Grading is done on four criteria (originality, versatility, harmony and rhythm, execution) in units of 0.1 points. The total K value of this flight is 240 K.

COMPOSING A FREE PROGRAM

While advance planning helps in all of the flights in each category, this is particularly true in the Free Program. Here the flown maneuvers are entirely at the discretion of the pilot, as long as he includes certain types of maneuvers. Since there are so many potential maneuvers and combinations of maneuvers, it is rare to see two identical sequences. If you do find two of the same it will usually be from people who fly together or from those wanting to imitate the success of a winner. The latter form of plagiarism is uncontrollable and usually doesn't make much difference, as Free Programs are usually "right" for only one plane-pilot combination.

The composers of the Known and Unknown Compulsory sequences are not necessarily benevolent individuals. They'll usually throw in a few twists that will be sure to challenge the pilots in that category and produce a spread in the scores. The Known Compulsory sequences used as illustrations earlier in this chapter all followed the basic rules of composition that we discussed before. Exit speeds and entry speeds were matched up and a certain amount of crosswind correction ability was built in. Aside from this, the sequences are expected to be flyable but challenging.

Since the Known and Unknown sequence composers aren't going to coddle you, you might as well take care of yourself in the Free Program. This assumes that you consider winning to be better than losing. If not, go on to the next section.

First, you must be able to fly the maneuvers. Not just do them, but do them well, so well that you are confident that you'll score well on each maneuver. If you can't do a good job on some maneuver in each of the types that must be included, then move down a category, for the other guys can. Some pilots in Intermediate and Advanced categories try to make their Free Programs into show pieces of their wide versatility and throw in a few maneuvers usually only seen in the higher categories. This is fine if you really do them well, but it usually doesn't work.

You also need to choose a sequence your airplane can fly. Altitude can be traded for entry speed just so many times before you reach the allowed minimum. Likewise, if your plane won't draw sustained vertical lines, you'd better leave out the double roll on a vertical line. In most cases you'll want to go out and test fly the sequence to see if it fits into the available altitude range. An underpowered airplane can compete above the Sportsman category, but it takes good planning as well as good flying. If there is any question about insufficient altitude, then you should try starting the sequence both fast and high. Be careful that when you convert that speed into altitude you don't break the upper altitude limit (3500 feet for all but Unlimited and 1000 meters for Unlimited). A good example of what not to do is to start a sequence with a Spin. In this case you bring little kinetic energy into the sequence and immediately lose altitude. Of course you can put an altitude gainer like the Immelmann right after, but you'll still end up lower than when you started the Spin and at a comparable airspeed. You've started losing altitude already. If you do several high entry speed maneuvers at the start and then put in the altitude gainer before that compulsory Spin, you will be ahead. This gives you fewer maneuvers to do while using up the available altitude. If you are blessed with an airplane that will do maneuver after maneuver without losing altitude, then you might as well get down to your lowest safe and allowable altitude and have at it. You can hide nothing from the judges down low, but your good maneuvers will get their best scores.

Dot your crosswind correction maneuvers throughout the sequence. By putting in several pairs of crosswind maneuvers at even spacings, you'll be relieved of the burden of putting in continuous crosswind correction on the individual maneuvers. Remember that what determines how far you are blown to the side is the time you have been flying, not how many maneuvers you have done. Rolls take much less time than Loops and you'll be blown off center less doing them; therefore, you can fit more of this type of maneuver between corrections.

Also consider the possibility of strong headwinds in composing a Free Program. The first maneuver of any flight sequence starts into the prevailing wind, so you will always be flying the same maneuver upwind or downwind. Since the natural tendency on low-power planes is to make the top of Square Loops too short, start that maneuver into the wind so that the same flight time will give a longer line on the top, which will be downwind. Likewise, it is very common to pinch Loops during the second half. By starting the Loop into the wind, the downwind on top will stretch the shape into a rounder form.

Wind should be considered in ordering the maneuvers and placing them in the aerobatic area. As we'll see in the next section, there is only a restricted volume in which to fly without penalty. Within this volume, the symmetry of placement of the maneuvers is important. If your airplane uses a high airspeed, a strong tail wind can easily blow you beyond the end boundary. It is better to leave out the downwind central maneuvers or put in fast ones like Rolls. Other maneuvers, such as the Reverse Half Cuban, are sometimes hard to fit in after a downwind central maneuver. There is no worse feeling than looking straight down on a downwind Hammerhead and watching the boundary slide past. Assume the wind is blowing something fierce when you make out your Free Program; you probably won't have to wait too long before you'll be glad you did.

A final guideline is to use all your possible maneuvers and keep them as simple as possible. The fact is, simple maneuvers are flown better than difficult maneuvers. If you put in 10 hard ones, instead of 20 easy ones, you'll probably not score as well, because your possible total points (determined by the maximum K value) will be no greater. Tiring at the end is not ordinarily a factor. Resist that temptation to put in the most impressive maneuvers you can do.

Let's examine a Free Program for the Unlimited category. In this case we have to begin and end in horizontal flight, have no more than 23 maneuvers and no more than 700 K. Maneuvers may not be repeated and must contain at least one from Aresti Families:

UNLIMITED · FREE
K=700

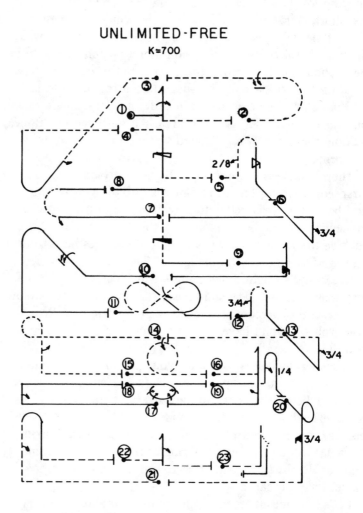

XIII-5

A Free Style program needs to include certain types of maneuvers and to be suited to the pilot and his airplane. This particular unlimited sequence is flown by the author to position well in the box and to involve minimum altitude loss.

4.1 (Upright Spins), 4.2 (Inverted Spins), 5.1 (Hammer-heads), 6 (Tailslides), 7.1–7.4 (Loops), 7.5–7.8 (Eights), 8.1 (Rolls), 8.2 (Point Rolls), 8.3.1 (Inside Snap Rolls), 8.3.2 (Outside Snap Rolls), 8.4 (Rolling Turn).

The sequence shown uses the maximum number of maneuvers and keeps the average difficulty factor down, recognizing that some of the required families have no low K maneuvers and some have no high K maneuvers that don't involve lots of altitude loss. It starts in the middle, where it is easy to be oriented and has three crosswind correction combinations and concentrates the slow maneuvers, such as the Loop and Hammerhead, in the upwind legs. Also important is that all of the crosswind combinations are placed on the upwind end of the aerobatic area. It uses simple maneuvers, which have a better chance of scoring well and all these maneuvers are no more difficult than those usually defining the Unlimited category. The 180 hp Pitts S1S will fly this sequence without serious loss of altitude since several climbing maneuvers followed by acceleration are used, compensating for the high entry speeds of other maneuvers.

THE AEROBATIC BOX

The maneuvers done in competition flying are to be flown in a restricted region known as the Box. Much easier said than done, for this volume can seem mighty small when you are trying to tie together a winning flight. Overhearing conversations in which pilots are talking about flying inside boxes has created confusion among the uninitiated more than once. We'll try to explain how this is a box without substance, unless you happen to be in it. The Box used for American competition is a square 3281 feet (1000 meters) on a side, with reference marks at the edges. The Box is actually defined by these 3281 feet

THE BOX

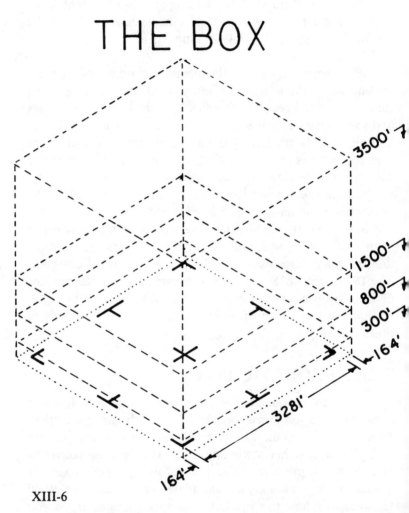

XIII-6

The Aerobatic Box is the volume in which competition maneuvers are flown. The edges and the top are the same for each category, but the bottom varies. Sportsman and Intermediate use 1500 feet, Advanced 800 feet and Unlimited 300 feet.

markings but has a 156 feet (50 meters) buffer around the edge. Since the pilot is concerned with the available space, he usually thinks in terms of a 3593-foot Box. Most flights have a left-right symmetry as viewed by the judges and this direction is called the X axis. All flights except the Four Minute Program are started on the X axis and into the wind. The Box has a ceiling of 3500 feet above the local terrain and a bottom determined category by category. For Sportsman and Intermediate the bottom is 1500 feet, Advanced, 800 feet and Unlimited, 300 feet. Although it is often argued that better flying would result from a larger box, this is just one of the added challenges that has to be accepted. From a safety point of view some argue that airplanes may be overstressed in trying to stay within the present Box. The alternate view is that a bigger Box would be used for obtaining higher airspeeds, with greater chance of overstressing than with the smaller Box and slower speeds. The primary reason for such a restricted Box is to allow good visibility by the judges; indeed, from their point of view it should be even lower, narrower and shorter. The near-best compromise is being approached, as small changes are being made from year to year. The judges are located on the extension of the Y axis, preferably at a distance of about 1000 feet, giving them a good view of the action. A final feature of the Box is the deadline, located anywhere from 500 feet from the edge of the Box, to within 500 feet of the crowd. Its intent is to prevent accidentally flying aerobatics over a populated area. If a contestant passes the deadline, he receives a score of 0 for that maneuver.

Boundary judges are located at as many corners as manpower allows. Deadline judges are at the ends of the deadline and whenever possible there should be one at each end, to allow accurate calls of such an important judgment. All of these judges use sighting aids.

POSITIONS

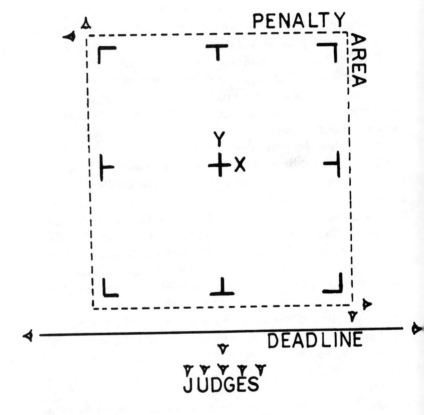

XIII-7

The Box is shown here as projected on the ground. The markings are placed just inside the penalty areas and judges (the all-seeing eyes) are located where they can best determine the quality of the maneuvers or the position of the airplane.

TRAFFIC CONTROL

Takeoff is controlled by a starter who is on the ground and usually near the downwind end of the active runway. Once the plane is airborne, entry into the Box is controlled by the chief judge. Radio use is not allowed, nor are radios available in many competition aircraft that are trying to keep their weight down. This means that ground direction of airplanes in flight must be used. Usually the chief judge controls a set of red and white panels located near or in the Box. These panels are large enough to be seen from the 3500 foot ceiling. Once it is determined that the judges are ready, a GO position (usually a white display) is given on the panels and the climbing aircraft is free to enter the Box. After he is in the Box, the panels are turned to STOP (usually solid red). This indicates that no new aircraft should enter, just in case the starter has someone else climbing for altitude while the previous pilot is doing his thing. If the climbing aircraft arrives at his starting altitude before he is given the GO sign, he goes into a holding pattern until it's his turn. In the event that there is danger to any aircraft in the air, a RECALL signal is given and everyone comes back and lands. Sometimes an itinerant aircraft flies through the Box or a competitor misses his cue and enters prematurely. This rarely happens, but when it does, the recall system needs to work. Sometimes this signal is a rapidly changing or mixed STOP/GO signal, but the best is a signal given in the middle of the Box. Traffic control is a vital safety feature in a contest. A measure of how well a contest is being run is how quickly the flights move, without compromising safety.

SCORING FLIGHTS

The whole equaling more than the sum of the parts, mathematically speaking is not correct but does describe the scoring of a competitor's flight. This is because there are more things that enter than the scores on individual maneuvers.

In chapter 12 we looked at the criteria for judging individual maneuvers. The judge uses these criteria to score the maneuvers one by one. This score, multiplied by the K factor, gives the number of points earned for that maneuver. This means that it's better to goof that 90° Turn (1 K) than the 360° Four Roll Turn (32 K). The sum of the points earned are added and form the base score from each judge.

There is one additional score given and that is for Positioning. This is an important one, as it has a K value of 10 for Sportsman, 15 for Intermediate and 25 for Advanced. It can earn you more points than some of the single maneuvers in any category. Positioning is evaluated on the basis of the symmetry and location of the maneuvers. It is there to allow scoring for how well the pilot places the maneuvers in the Box and compensates for the prevailing wind conditions. It is a qualitative score, judged on how well the pilot centered the mid-Box maneuvers, located the end-Box maneuvers at similar distances on both ends and placed the maneuvers along the Y axis. It is not uncommon to see flights in a strong headwind (along the X axis) locate every maneuver on the downwind side of the Box and, of course, these flights get low Positioning scores.

After the individual judges base scores are added, a number of subtractions may be necessary. If the boundaries of the Box were crossed, points will be subtracted. If a pilot flew too high or low, he'll be penalized, and if he flies too much beneath the Box, the entire flight will be given a 0. Obviously, any maneuver that was omitted will be given a 0, but so will maneuvers flown out of order or in the wrong direction. There was the case of an outstanding competitor who entered the Box in the wrong direction, flew everything backwards, and received all 0's for an otherwise beautiful flight.

After these corrections are applied, the total points are calculated for each judge and then the highest and lowest judges' total are thrown out and the remaining three scores are used to determine the overall total for that contestant's flight. Throwing out the high and low is intended to correct for judges who consistently judge one contestant very differently from the other judges. It is a step in the right direction; however, it does not allow for the judge who consistently grades *all* contestants either high or low. A new system of score adjustment developed in Germany, called the Bauer system, takes the individual judge's scores and performs elaborate mathematical calculations, which bring everyone's scores into line. It does not distort the intent of scores and does allow for systematic differences between individual judges. It is recommended at contests with categories having at least seven judges and twenty pilots, otherwise it does not give meaningful statistics. One must be aware of the sad tale of the statistician who drowned in the river that was on the average only six inches deep! Since most score calculations are done by mini-computers at the contest, the Bauer system is easily used. The only disadvantage—you don't know your score until everyone in your category has flown and some anonymous computer is changing your score by a method most pilots don't understand.

14
Contest Flying
—What It's Like

AEROBATIC CONTESTS are great—even better when you win something. They are opportunities for people of similar interests to get together and swap tales and facts and to fly and see flying done. If you're looking for a spectator sport, you'd better stay at home, because there is a job for everyone. The end result of a summer contest is usually some useful new technical fact, a determination to get more practice before the next time, possibly a trophy and undoubtedly a sunburn. You start early, end late, work yourself into a state of nervous anticipation and generally have a good time. Throughout this variety of activities there flows the current of intense competition—competition between pilots and competition of pilots against their own standards and goals. In this chapter we'll participate in one day of a typical contest and even take a competition flight.

A TYPICAL CONTEST DAY

It starts in the early morning, with a little mist in the air and red-jacket-clad participants standing around trying to wake up.

194

In the main hangar a handful of owners are trying to locate their birds and figure out how to get them out, for the airplanes were stacked incredibly tight the night before. The chief judge barks out the call for the contest briefing with the roll call of the pilots, judges and judges' staffs. Obviously, he was formerly a member of the military, rumored to be a retired colonel, but sounds more like a drill sergeant as he marches down the rolls and gets those inevitable stragglers moving faster into hearing distance. He then quickly moves through the checklist, describing which categories will fly that day and in which order, which pilots will fly, announces the direction of flight based on the present and predicted winds and the traffic control procedures. Most of the men and women hearing their day being dictated have done this all before, but there are a few first timers and they feel just a little confused by the seeming disorder. By the end of the day they'll appreciate the detailed orchestration that has gone into those plans being described.

Almost all of those who will be flying today arrived the day before. They come singly and in pairs and all do a lot of stretching once they get out, for aerobatic airplanes are not designed with pilot comfort in mind. Most of the pilots come from within a few hundred miles of the contest location, but there are always a few who have had to make the trip in a number of legs. They can usually be spotted by the way they climb out. Once unlimbered, all register with the contest organizers, showing proof of their legal status as pilots and the integrity of their aircraft. The Box will have been open and each arrival is allowed at least one practice session in the Box to get a feel for where the landmarks are and determine what they will use as references the next day.

The briefing is over now and the contest chairman deploys his troops. Boundary judges to their stations, starters to the flight line and judging teams to the judges' line. All these people are tied together into a unit by portable radios, so that activities can be coordinated. There is also a set of runners who will collect score sheets and, later, bring food and beverages to those not rotating off their assignments. The score computers will have already programmed their calculators and will await those first score sheets.

These people share an interest in aviation (to be sure, in some cases, it is aviators) and will be working very hard at the sport. Some participants will have had to satisfy conditions of training and experience, like the judges, in order to qualify for their assignments while others will bring nothing but enthusiasm to their jobs. All of this is brought about by the local hosts, who put in many hours preparing for a smoothly run contest.

The pilots who are flying in the first category heard their flight order called during the briefing and line up their planes behind the starter. However, the first pilot in the air will not be a competitor. A non-competitor is usually selected to "fly the lines." This is done after the judging teams are in position in order to allow the judges to see where the edges of the Box are located and how an airplane looks when flying at the bottom of the Box.

While all of this is being done, a rather strange ritual is being performed on the flight line. Each pilot prepares for his flight in his own fashion, from quiet contemplation to animated pacing—and everything in-between. The strangest part is the "Dance of the Aerobat." Even though the sequence may have been practiced dozens of times, everyone seems to think that going through it one more time can't hurt. Usually this is done with the flat hand simulating the airplane and closely observing the boundaries of an imaginary Box projected on the asphalt. Climbs, Dives, Rolls and Spins are all done in silent progression as the pilot walks, turns and pirouettes in a pattern that carries him through the flight that he soon will make. Filmed from a distance and put to music, the dance has acquired its name to the amusement of almost everyone.

The first competitor into the Box has the advantage of a short wait but the disadvantage of being the wind dummy. A certain added challenge is heaped on this pilot, but it's the luck of the draw. Once he's in the Box, the contest usually proceeds smoothly, with airplanes in the Box much of the time, spread out only by the time needed to sort the scores for the previous pilot who may have gone low or flown some maneuver in the wrong direction. The intervals are usually a little longer between the Free Programs since the judge and his caller need to be sure that they know what to expect in the next flight.

Flight follows flight until each category is finished, succeeded by the next, with some changes of judging personnel, for a judge in one category may be a contestant in another. The day gets hotter, the sun moves in the sky and a pattern of activity is established, punctuated only by the occasional encroaching itinerant airplane or low cloud. Since the weather tomorrow may be worse than today's, the flying is usually continued as long as possible into the evening.

The airplanes are there in the air and can be watched by anyone. Some pilots will watch their competitors and others will not. What they all watch is the scoreboard. How you feel about your flight may not be related to what the judges thought, especially if you left something out! The score sheets, with the judges' comments, will be available to each pilot; this is the only way of finding out what the judges want to see.

The Sportsman pilot watches the Unlimited competitor's flight with a mixture of awe and challenge, perhaps wondering if he'll ever be there. The Unlimited pilot watches the Sportsman competitor and appreciates how hard it is to do these maneuvers well in a low-powered airplane and how hard it can be when you're just getting started. This is an aerobatic happening and they are all part of it, whether it is a local weekend contest or one of the week-long national events in Fond du Lac, Wisconsin, or Sherman, Texas.

A FLIGHT

I sit in the cockpit, baking, waiting and convincing myself that I am ready. Everything that can be done has been done, and the only thing left is the flying. Last evening at the banquet the Advanced Unknown's were distributed, which made the evening a little bit less festive for me, although the other pilots seemed to enjoy themselves all the more after that. I noticed the others who had received Unknowns heading off on their own instead of hanging around, and did the same. It can be flown —can't it? My silent response had been, "Oh my gosh, I've never done one of these," a sentiment echoed out loud by others on first examination, when they saw that Outside Spin from Upright. Then the sequence was taken apart maneuver by maneuver and as a sequence. What altitude should be used? If I start too high, I lose power and it is harder to judge. If I start too low, I may find myself on the bottom of the Box flying at entry speeds too slow to do the maneuvers well. The crosswind maneuvers were studied. If the wind is from the right on maneuver 1, then I'll need to roll left on number 2 to come out upright and then roll right in number 4 to come out inverted into the wind, etc. Finally, I drew the sequence on a chart, which now appears before me on the instrument panel. I used a color code, with all downwind maneuvers drawn in red, just in case I get lost and need to reorient myself.

I am calm. I am ready. I have watched the clouds drift by and predicted the wind's effect when I fly. It's going to be quartering from the right on the first maneuver but not too strong, so I'll have to do number 7 into the wind and number 10 downwind across the Box. I am calm, but why did that photographer have to get so damned close when I was hand-flying through the sequence just before climbing in? I am calm. After all, no one is making me do this; I'm strictly a volunteer, doing this because I want to. Boy, it's hot. If I pick up 300 points, I can probably move up two places. Looking up I see someone entering the Box. He overrotated the spin and zeroed it! That was the leader and that was the maneuver I've only read about. Where does that leave me? I *am* calm. Were those people talking to me as I pushed the plane out?

The starter gives the signal, and a competitor from another category pulls the prop through while I prime the engine. Look at that, it started on the first hot blade. Good omen? I taxi out, swinging the nose left and right. I can see ahead around that big Lycoming engine and describe a continuous S path along the taxiway. There's the flagman and I hold short of the runway. The run-up on the engine seems normal, and I give the lap belts a final pull so they are as tight as can be. The shoulder restraints are snug but not tight. I see the present competitor cross overhead; he has obviously finished his flight, and I get the go ahead from the flagman and am off.

I add full power and then forward stick. Once it's rolling the Pitts really accelerates, and I lift off as the airspeed passes through 70 mph after only 500 feet of runway. I want the maximum rate of climb off the deck so I use 90 mph at the start. Let the nose down to allow the airspeed to build up, which gives me more time to get oriented and keep the cylinder temperature down. I've got five minutes to climb and even now should only use a small fraction to get the 2300 feet I figured that I need. The panels are red. The judges must be having a conference on that last flight. It's a beautiful day. You can see forever. Climb parallel to the X and Y axis to see how the wind really is. Good. Looks like I can use the turn directions I figured out on the ground. There go the panels; it's my turn.

I turn in to the Box and line up with the Y axis a quarter mile out and give two dips of the wing to tell the judges this is for score. I can imagine the alert of "Heads Up" being given on the judges' line. If I do the Spin before I get in the Box, it's a 0 even if perfect, so I'd better make sure it's in. Pull the power off and the airplane slows, then I reverse the controls as it's supposed to be done, just at the stall. The nose drops through and the autorotation starts. Stop it on heading with a touch of opposite rudder. Hot dog—made it. Draw the vertical line and build up plenty of speed to get 150 at the bottom. Pull five G's for the first vertical up line, Quarter Roll left, then hold the vertical as

ADVANCED UNKNOWN

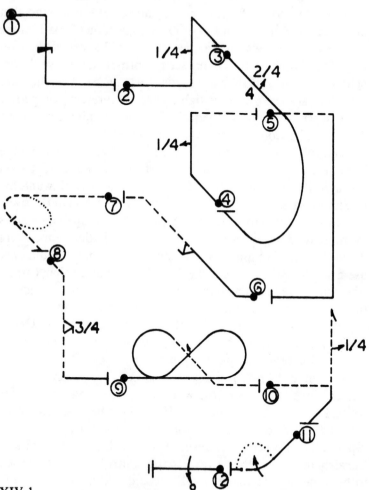

XIV-1

The Advanced Unknown Flight sequence described in the text is given here in its Aresti notation.

long as I can and still have flying speed, slowly push over to upright, with lots of right rudder to keep on heading. Here comes maneuver 3, the Split S with a hesitation at knife-edge. I roll inverted with a point and pull into the Split S. Staring at the ground, I can see that I put the Spin too late, for I'm past center. Too late now. Not too tight; I need the 150 again. Into number 4, Quarter Roll right then pull over to the inverted. Keep it flat and slow to the end of the Box then down into the Half Square Loop. Five G's at the bottom. Going from minus one G to plus five does make a difference, a little gray there at the bottom. I pull up into maneuver number 6 with the climbing 45° line, and damn! I oversnapped the Half Snap Roll but took it out very slowly. I wonder how much the judges thought it was. I try to draw an equal length line, then pull over into inverted level flight. Turn right into the wind, with lots of bank, and drive over to the upwind side of the Box before pulling down for the Three Quarter Snap on a vertical line, which is maneuver number 8. Let's see, I want to turn right so I snap left. I undersnapped and they probably saw me aileron it onto heading; I was also quite positive after. I drive into the wind for the Horizontal Eight. Pull up and over, hit the line, half roll upright, hit the line then pull for the second half, then let it float down to the inverted 45° and hold it until I'm sure of coming out at the original altitude. The judges can peg that altitude very closely. Out inverted and here comes the end of the Box. Push hard to about minus four G's till we're straight up for the Hammerhead. That doesn't feel any more comfortable than the first time I did one. Evidently the lap belts have loosened because I was really hanging out on them. Hope I did it right, because I can't see anything of the Box as I'm on the end with my head pointed out. Kick the rudder on the top, then set the vertical line, Quarter Roll left and pull out pointed at the judges' side, and drive just far enough to be sure I can Barrel Roll to the left. Maneuver 11 is a rolling turn to the left along the judges' line. After that I'm immediately into the Barrel Roll. It's not too smooth and beyond the center at inverted but not too bad either. Another pair of wing dips and I'm done. That has to be the busiest three and a half minutes of my life. Now to see if I can land this thing without adding insult to injury.

Taxi in, shut down the engine and take a big breath. I'm not really tired but something has been taken out. I look around at my friends and see if their expressions say I've botched something badly and didn't know it, then put the plane away and start waiting. The scores are finally posted and it looks like it wasn't too bad. Those points may be picked up. Finally, they're all in, and I've finished in the money (figuratively speaking). That's great; it's not like winning it all, but it sure beats a punch in the nose.

It doesn't always end this well, just frequently enough to keep you coming back to try again. Even in not winning there can be pride, for think of how many aerobatic pilots talk a good flight but never seem to make it out in front of the judges. Even when you feel like one of those Trojan soldiers who came home on their shields, there is always another chance. As one competitor was heard to say at Fond du Lac, "Well, guess I'll head for home, lick my wounds and practice for the Nationals, for if you will not risk failure, you will surely surrender success."

15
Epilogue

THERE IS A TRUE SAYING about life that "none of us are going to get out of this alive." Every mature individual recognizes his personal mortality and values life for its meaning and worth. Within this perspective, he learns and teaches, works and plays. All these activities are ones that are meaningful to him; for many of us, aerobatic flying is an integral part of our lives. It is not without risk. The experienced aerobatic pilot will have passed the stage of apprehension that he may have felt at the beginning of his training, but the recognition of risk is always there. Unfortunately, each year there are a few accidents and when someone you know has one, then the reality of risk becomes very clear. Each accident carries a lesson. Not a message to desist, go home and vegetate, but a lesson on what to do and not to do, and how to safely pursue aerobatics.

Friends now gone have left messages. Don't push your skills and experience beyond their limits. Build, but build slowly, in small steps and from a firm foundation. Personally know your equipment and never fly if there is any question of the aircraft's integrity. Resist the temptation to fly for someone else. Always choose your altitude, time and maneuvers as if no one would ever know that you flew—except you. These survival rules apply in all circumstances, especially if there is a crowd watching. I would rather not have learned these things in the way that I have, but it makes the messages more real.

The keys to safety are knowledge and discipline. Knowledge comes only with experience and thought; this is where the proper training and approach become important. Each new experience in aerobatics must be fit into the knowledge derived from previous experiences. If you don't understand what happened and were just an interested spectator, you will not have learned. Don't push yourself into new flight regimes that are dangerous for you. There are challenges enough; don't worry about running out of them. The excellent safety record of modern organized competition reflects the positive results of progressive development of pilots by working up through the categories.

Discipline is the other key and the one that is more obvious when ignored. Discipline begins when you are building your aircraft and you take the extra time and care to make sure each part is just right. It applies similarly when you are inspecting an airplane for purchase and have to say no because you don't like its history, even though the cashier's check is there in your pocket, it's a bargain, you've come for the inspection with a one-way airline ticket and there just aren't very many planes of that model on the market. Discipline extends through the preflight inspection, selecting practice areas and setting minimum altitudes for specific maneuvers. Discipline also applies while you are flying, through setting a fixed number of turns for that flat spin, determining to break off a maneuver when it's not going right and not flying for anyone except yourself. If you think this emphasis on discipline makes for a dull sport pursued by a bunch of dull people, you obviously haven't seen good aerobatic flying or met the pilots at an aerobatic contest!

In the introductory chapter I talked about the reasons for learning and for performing aerobatics. The reasons for learning aerobatics are important (safety, skill, efficiency), but these are separate from the reasons for doing aerobatics over a sustained period. Aerobatics are an endless challenge: there is always something to be learned and to be tried. Aerobatics are a form of poetry and grace, the pursuit of a perfect expression which is not recorded except in memory.

Aerobatics are an extension of ourselves into a free environment that is available to all who wish to enter.

Glossary

Adverse Yaw A force caused by the downward ailerons having more drag than the upward ailerons. This factor becomes important in executing coordinated turns and precise rolls.

Aerobatics Flight of an aircraft in a manner assuming unusual attitudes while performing well-defined maneuvers.

Ailerons Hinged portions of the outer trailing edges of a wing. When moved opposite to one another, they add or subtract lift from the wing, producing roll.

Angle of Attack The angle at which a wing meets the air.

Attitude The direction an aircraft is pointed.

Autorotation A stable flight condition in which differential lift of the wings produces continuous rotation of the aircraft.

Bank The angle the wings make during a turn or roll.

Elevator Hinged portion of the horizontal stabilizer. When moved, it adds or subtracts lift from the tail, changing the pitch attitude.

G The unit used for the load factor.

Heading The direction an aircraft is pointed across the earth's surface.

Horizontal Stabilizer A small wing section attached to the tail of an aircraft to control the balance.

Incidence The angle at which the wings are attached to an aircraft.

Load Factor The ratio of the apparent weight to the true weight of an aircraft.

P-factor The yawing force caused when the propeller is rotating about an axis at a large angle to the direction of flight.

Pitch The attitude of an aircraft as the nose moves up and down.

Pitot The primary sensor of the airspeed indicator.

Precession The force that results when trying to push against a spinning object.

Roll The motion of an aircraft around a line through its middle.

Rudder A hinged vertical portion of the tail that changes the heading of the aircraft.

Spin Autorotation at low or zero forward speed.

Stall The condition in which the angle of attack exceeds that for the maximum amount of lift.

Torque A force, applied to an object, that produces rotation.

Track The path of an aircraft in flight. ˙

Yaw Motion about a perpendicular line through the center of an aircraft.

Index